Your
A.W.E.S.O.M.E.
Life

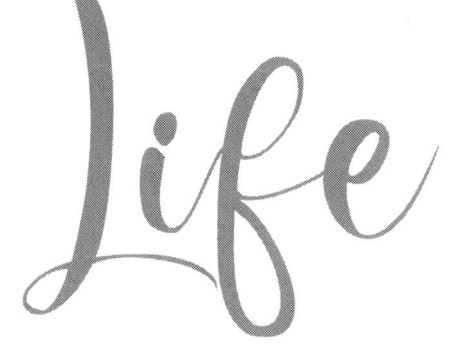

How to
Reach Your Healthy Weight and
Live Your Life Feeling Energized and Balanced

MARGARET LEDANE

Copyright © 2018 by Margaret Clark LeDane

Your A.W.E.S.O.M.E. Life: How to Reach Your Healthy Weight and Live Your Life Feeling Energized and Balanced

by Margaret Clark LeDane, CHC

All rights reserved. No part of this book may be reproduced or transmitted in any form or by any means, electronic or mechanical, including photocopying, recording or by any informational and retrieval system without written permission from the author, except for the inclusion of brief quotations and / or show brief video clips in a review.

Disclaimer: The author of this book does not dispense medical or psychological advice or prescribe the use of any technique as a form of treatment for physical, medical or emotional problems without the advice of a physician, either directly or indirectly. The intent of the author is only to offer information of a general nature to help you in your pursuit of a healthier life. In the event that you use any of the information in this book for yourself, which is your constitutional right, the author and the publisher assume no responsibility for your actions.

CONTENTS

ACKNOWLEDGEMENTS 7

INTRODUCTION. 9

**THE FIRST SECRET TO FINDING YOUR
A.W.E.S.O.M.E. IS CREATING AN
ACTIVE MIND AND BODY.** **15**

KEY #1 TO HAVING AN ACTIVE MIND AND BODY
IS KEEPING YOUR BRAIN ALIVE. 15

KEY #2 TO HAVING AN ACTIVE MIND AND BODY
IS KEEPING YOUR RELATIONSHIPS HEALTHY. 18

KEY #3 TO HAVING AN ACTIVE MIND AND BODY
IS ENJOYING YOUR CHILDREN! 26

KEY #4 TO HAVING AN ACTIVE MIND AND BODY
IS PARTICIPATING AND VOLUNTEERING IN
YOUR COMMUNITIES! 28

KEY #5 TO HAVING AN ACTIVE MIND AND BODY
IS JOINING A CLUB! 31

KEY #6 TO HAVING AN ACTIVE MIND AND BODY
IS COOKING! 32

KEY #7 TO HAVING AN ACTIVE MIND AND BODY
IS SAYING NO! 34

THE SECOND SECRET TO FINDING YOUR A.W.E.S.O.M.E. IS EATING WHOLESOME FOODS! 36

FOOD #1 IN WHOLESOME FOODS IS VEGETABLES (OF COURSE!)........................... 37

FOOD #2 IN WHOLESOME FOODS IS FRUIT!............. 40

FOOD #3 IN WHOLESOME FOODS ARE ORGANIC NON-GMO GRAINS!...................................... 42

FOOD #4 IN WHOLESOME FOODS IS PROTEIN!.......... 45

FOOD #5 IN WHOLESOME FOODS IS SUGAR!............ 48

FOOD #6 IN WHOLESOME FOODS IS FAT! 51

FOOD #6 IN WHOLESOME FOODS IS WATER!............ 54

FOOD #7 IN WHOLESOME FOODS IS CONDIMENTS AND SPICES!............................. 58

THE THIRD SECRET TO FINDING YOUR A.W.E.S.O.M.E. IS EXERCISING! 60

BENEFIT #1 IN EXERCISE IS HEART HEALTH! 60

BENEFIT #2 IN EXERCISE IS BONE HEALTH!............. 61

BENEFIT #3 IN EXERCISE IS CALORIE HEALTH! 62

BENEFIT #4 IN EXERCISE IS SUGAR HEALTH!............ 63

BENEFIT #5 IN EXERCISE IS FRIEND / PARTNER / ME TIME!.. 65

BENEFIT #6 IN EXERCISE IS BRAIN HEALTH! 66

BENEFIT #7 IN EXERCISE IS EXAMPLE SETTING! 67

THE FOURTH SECRET TO FINDING YOUR A.W.E.S.O.M.E. IS SLEEPING! 71

BENEFIT #1 FOR SLEEPING IS A SUPERCHARGED IMMUNE SYSTEM!....................................... 73

BENEFIT #2 FOR SLEEPING IS GROWING! 73
BENEFIT #3 FOR SLEEPING IS BRAIN HEALTH! 75
BENEFIT #4 FOR SLEEPING IS BEAUTY SLEEP!........... 76
BENEFIT #5 FOR SLEEPING IS REDUCED HUNGER! 77
BENEFIT #6 FOR SLEEPING IS RELAXATION!............. 78

**THE FIFTH SECRET TO FINDING YOUR
A.W.E.S.O.M.E. IS ORGANIZATION! 81**

AREA #1 FOR ORGANIZATION IS YOUR PANTRY! 82
AREA #2 FOR ORGANIZATION IS YOUR FREEZER! 83
AREA #3 FOR ORGANIZATION IS YOUR REFRIGERATOR!. 84
AREA #4 FOR ORGANIZATION IS USING AN
ONLINE CALENDAR!.................................... 86
AREA #5 FOR ORGANIZATION IS STORAGE
ROOMS, CLOSETS, KITCHEN CABINETS AND GARAGE!.. 87
AREA #6 FOR ORGANIZATION IS LISTS AND OFFICES!... 89
AREA #7 FOR ORGANIZATION IS MEALS!................ 91

**THE SIXTH SECRET TO FINDING YOUR
A.W.E.S.O.M.E. IS BEING MINDFUL!..................... 94**

STEP #1 FOR BEING MINDFUL IS FORGETTING
THE SMALL STUFF!..................................... 94
STEP #2 FOR BEING MINDFUL IS IGNORING
GOSSIP AND DRAMA!................................... 95
STEP #3 FOR BEING MINDFUL IS PICKING A
MANTRA (OR TWO)! 97
STEP #4 FOR BEING MINDFUL IS CHANGING
COURSE WHEN HEADING FOR THE REFRIGERATOR! ... 98
STEP #5 FOR BEING MINDFUL IS BEING THANKFUL! 99

STEP #6 FOR BEING MINDFUL IS SEEKING HELP
FOR DEPRESSION! 100

STEP #7 FOR BEING MINDFUL IS LAUGHTER! 102

STEP #8 FOR BEING MINDFUL IS BEING POSITIVE! 103

STEP #9 FOR BEING MINDFUL IS NOT TO WORRY! 104

**THE SEVENTH SECRET TO FINDING YOUR
A.W.E.S.O.M.E. IS ENVISIONING AND LIVING
YOUR TRUE LIFE! 107**

STEP #1 FOR ENVISIONING AND LIVING YOUR
TRUE LIFE IS LOOKING AT YOUR PHYSICAL SELF! 107

STEP #2 FOR ENVISIONING AND LIVING YOUR
TRUE LIFE IS BEING HAPPY WITH YOUR
PHYSICAL SURROUNDINGS! 109

STEP #3 FOR ENVISIONING AND LIVING YOUR
TRUE LIFE IS CLOSELY EXAMINING YOUR
RELATIONSHIP WITH YOUR SPOUSE OR PARTNER! 110

STEP #4 FOR ENVISIONING AND LIVING YOUR
TRUE LIFE IS EXAMINING YOUR CAREER! 112

STEP #5 FOR ENVISIONING AND LIVING YOUR
TRUE LIFE IS TRAVELING! 113

STEP # 6 FOR ENVISIONING AND LIVING YOUR
TRUE LIFE IS EXAMINING YOUR RELIGIOUS
BELIEFS OR SPIRITUALITY! 115

SUMMARY 123

ABOUT THE AUTHOR 124

SPECIAL OFFER FROM MARGARET! 125

ACKNOWLEDGEMENTS

I am deeply appreciative of my amazing parents, Carlotta and Preston Clark for raising me with the belief that hard work, independent thinking, and perseverance will get you wherever you want to go. They allowed me to learn from my own mistakes while providing me the support to improve and continue.

Thank you to my sister, Miriam and my brother in law, Matt for their love, support and influence on my life.

Thank you to my children, Clark and Julia who are truly awesome teens.

Thank you to all the people who've allowed me to coach them over the years, family, friends and clients. I've learned so much from you.

Lastly, I would like to thank my wonderful partner Stephen for all of his help and support over these last years. Thanks Match.com for bringing Scardy22 and HockeyMom1907 together, all those years ago.

INTRODUCTION

I wanted to feel A.W.E.S.O.M.E. again...and I didn't know how. How do I get rid of the "baby weight" (now that my babies are walking, talking and, well, driving) and ditch the mom jeans once and for all? Why did I allow myself to balloon to this unhealthy size? How do I get the weight off and keep it off for good? How do I gain energy and find emotional freedom and balance? I'm done being a yo-yo. I want to BE healthy and FEEL healthy. I want to LOOK GOOD! Where do I start?

It is no fun feeling this way. But the good news is you don't have to feel this way! Here's my story and how you can avoid my mistakes and enjoy my successes. I figured out how to feel A.W.E.S.O.M.E., and I'm so happy that I can share it with you.

When I got pregnant the first time, I was ecstatic. I wanted two children and I was on my way. The strange thing, looking back, was that I think I was ecstatic for two reasons. The first reason was my new bundle of joy growing so happily inside of me, and the second reason was that I could eat whatever and whenever I wanted...something I had been dying to do since puberty.

Puberty for me was when all hell broke loose. My body started to grow and move in all sorts of directions and all of a sudden I had to...heaven forbid...watch my weight. I had never had to watch my weight. What's going on? How completely annoying!

As a teen and until college, and I stress until college, I did a pretty good job of staying a healthy weight, which was probably due to my athletics. I'm pretty sure if I weren't as active as I was, my weight would have been a huge problem.

I loved to dance and I usually did that three times a week, and I played school sports. Through my middle and high school years at 5'9", I stayed around 145 pounds. I realize NOW that I probably looked pretty good. Young athletes have a lot of muscle, so even though I wasn't a stick like most of my friends (why are best friends always sticks?), I was a healthy weight. Don't get me wrong, this took a lot of work to stay at this weight and I always felt fat.

Not to bore you too much with my fluctuations during college, but let's just say at one time the college 15 was the college 25. Yo-yoing over the next ten years and you're now caught up to... pregnancy.

So, eating, eating and more eating...that's what I did. After all, I was pregnant so who would notice my weight gain? When I got on the scale at the doctor checkups it was all baby weight, right? If my belly was going to grow, then why not have the rest of me grow, too? Didn't they have to match? Wouldn't I look out of proportion if they didn't?

So I didn't worry about the weight gain until the day I proudly brought my son home, got on the scale and, gulp, read 210! Holy guacamole, I just had a 10-pound baby. Shouldn't more have come off during my 24 hours of killer childbirth?

I mean, really, 24 hours of intense pain, pain so bad that you swear there's someone hiding under the bed jabbing a knife in your side as soon as you close your eyes for a half of a second hoping to either die or get that demon out of you. With that kind of pain shouldn't I have burned off at least...25 pounds? Isn't that the way it works? Well, not so much.

So those "few" pounds (plus the 10 extra with which I started) were definitely my nemesis. What to do? How can I possibly lose the weight? I'm a new mother, so does it really matter? My husband doesn't care, my baby doesn't care, so why do I care? Maybe I don't. I'm quite comfortable in these maternity clothes. After all, I really haven't gotten my money's worth out of them. They're stretchy; they wash and dry with ease. So why not just stay in them for a while? Why did I have so many excuses when I knew in my soul that I wanted to feel A.W.E.S.O.M.E. again? And currently at 210, I did not!

Over the next year I tried to exercise and eat right, and eventually I did lose some weight. But that still left me at a, well, hefty 180.

So when my son was 13 months old, I became pregnant a second time. Great. Ecstatic a second time, because you guessed it, one my new baby and two I can EAT – A LOT. So off I go, but this time starting at my newfound weight of 180. I'm pretty sure I stopped looking at the scale in the doctor's office somewhere around five months. I just wanted to enjoy my last pregnancy and I was, well, horrified too. I've repressed the final scale memory, but we'll just say…245…ish! It was ugly, very, very ugly.

Now, don't get me wrong, my children are fabulous and I wouldn't return them for the world, especially for my near perfect (wishful thinking), pre-baby booty, but I will not resign myself to a life of stretchy pants either. So, what to do? I started walking and not eating everything in sight and I lost some weight over the years. But I never got down to an A.W.E.S.O.M.E. healthy weight…one that I had experienced before children and one that I wanted to experience again.

I went up and down and stayed a good 30 pounds over where I wanted to be and where it was healthy for me to be. I stress healthy because my blood pressure stayed on the high normal side with the extra weight. Once the weight came off and my exercise routine stayed consistent, my blood pressure dropped dramatically and it now stays in the completely low normal range.

So why did I stay stuck for so very long? Well, I didn't know what to do and I felt overwhelmed by which 'diet' was right for me. 'Diet' a word that I hate as a verb, but a word that I love as a noun.

A diet of clean food is crucial for living at a healthy weight, but dieting is for the birds.

No one should ever have to diet if their lifestyle is full of healthy habits and excellent nutrition.

OK, so now you know my history, pain and frustrations, so let's move on to the fun part – how to find your A.W.E.S.O.M.E.

I want YOU to benefit from my mistakes by learning from my successes. I'm not going to go into the science behind certain foods, but I will share with you the importance of certain foods in your diet.

This book should be a quick, fun read and something to which you can refer for years. After all, sometimes your clothes get a little tight occasionally. Especially during the Thanksgiving / Christmas "grazing all day" time of year. The number one New Year's resolution...drum roll please...LOSE WEIGHT AND GET IN SHAPE. OK, let's do it!

Here are your 7 A.W.E.S.O.M.E. Secrets:

1) A = Active Mind and Body
    Key #1 – Keep Your Brain Alive
    Key #2 – Keep Your Relationships Healthy
    Key #3 – Enjoy Your Children
    Key #4 – Get Involved in Your Community
    Key #5 – Join a Club
    Key #6 – Cook
    Key #7 – Say NO
2) W = Wholesome Foods
    Food #1 – Vegetables
    Food #2 – Fruit
    Food #3 – Whole Grains
    Food #4 – Protein
    Food #5 – Sugar
    Food #6 – Fat
    Food #7 – Water
    Food #8 – Condiments

3) E = Exercise
    Benefit #1 – Heart Health
    Benefit #2 – Bone Health
    Benefit #3 – Brain Health
    Benefit #4 – Calorie Health
    Benefit #5 – Sugar Health
    Benefit #6 – Friend / Partner / Me Time
    Benefit #7 – Example Setting
4) S = Sleep
    Benefit #1 – Supercharged Immune System
    Benefit #2 – Growing
    Benefit #3 – Brain Health
    Benefit #4 – Beauty Sleep
    Benefit #5 – Reduced Hunger
    Benefit #6 – Relaxation
5) O = Organization
    Idea #1 – Pantry
    Idea #2 – Freezer
    Idea #3 – Refrigerator
    Idea #4 – Calendar
    Idea #5 – Storage Rooms and Closets
    Idea #6 – Lists
    Idea #7 – Meals
6) M = Mindful
    Step #1 – Forgetting the Small Stuff
    Step #2 – Ignoring Gossip and Drama
    Step #3 – Picking a Mantra
    Step #4 – Changing Course when Heading
        for the Refrigerator
    Step #5 – Being Thankful
    Step #6 – Seeking Help for Depression
    Step #7 – Laughing

          Step #8 – Being Positive
          Step #9 – Not Worrying
7)   E = Envisioning and Enjoying Your True Life
          Step #1 – Looking at Your Physical Self
          Step #2 – Being Happy with Your
                    Physical Surroundings
          Step #3 – Closely Examining Your Relationship
                    with your Spouse or Partner
          Step #4 – Examining Your Career
          Step #5 – Traveling
          Step #6 – Examining Your Religious
                    Beliefs and Spirituality

OK, let's start working on these secrets…

THE FIRST SECRET TO FINDING YOUR A.W.E.S.O.M.E. IS CREATING AN ACTIVE MIND AND BODY.

My very basic rule for this journey is, you cannot have a healthy body without having a healthy mind. I'll repeat that. You cannot have a healthy body without having a healthy mind. Put that in stone. Your success depends on that combination. To create a healthy mind it must be active. To create a healthy body it must be active. Let's begin...

KEY #1

TO HAVING AN ACTIVE MIND AND BODY IS KEEPING YOUR BRAIN ALIVE.

One way to do this is by having a spicy life. No, I don't mean for you and your husband to swing with your neighbors. (Although I've heard it's common in some neighborhoods:)) I mean, getting out of your loving family's everyday necessary routine, and putting some fun stuff on your calendar. Spice it up. Make it sizzle!

You need time for:

1) you (no partner or children)
2) you + partner (no children)
3) family

Even if you are divorced and dating, you still need the trifecta as I'll call it, or you won't have the balance that is needed to keep your brain alive. And remember, keeping your brain alive is key number one to having an active mind and body. And an active mind and body is Step 1 to feeling A.W.E.S.O.M.E. Here are some examples of how to spice it up and keep that brain alive.

What can I do for me time?

- Volunteer at your church
- Join your local Junior League
- Work one night a week at your favorite store (you get the discount and you meet new people)
- Find a gym partner
- Take an art class at the local college or at the local rec center
- Learn a new language
- Do crossword puzzles
- Take a dance class – ballet, tap, jazz, salsa, hip hop, Zumba
- Join a book club
- Sign up for a 5k or more. It will make you train.
- Take a bath with a Do Not Disturb sign on the door. Read a book. Light up the mind while relaxing. Or, just plain relax and meditate.
- Take a cooking class
- Go to a chick flick
- Take a walk

- Go to yoga
- Shop

What can I do with my partner? (Other than that...but including that.)

- Dinner date. This is my favorite because not only is the food and atmosphere relaxing, but it gives you hours of uninterrupted time to talk. Communication is a huge component to a good marriage.
- Go out with another couple. Laughter and memories help seal a good relationship.
- Take a walk
- Go to yoga
- Take dance lessons
- Lift weights at the gym
- Sign up for a 5k
- Take cooking class
- Find a sport you both like – tennis, bowling, biking, golf, boating, sailing, hiking
- Sex. Yes, it is important and not once a month. Try for at least once a week.

What can we do as a family?

- Biking
- Hiking
- Beach boardwalk games
- Board games
- Wii games
- Cards
- Museum
- Movie

- Go to the beach
- Rake leaves
- Walk the dog
- Go shopping and eat out
- Play ball in the yard
- Go to a local festival

There are endless possibilities. What's your passion? Find it and go with it. You'll be surprised by how a small outlet can be so uplifting. It's not only the outlet, but looking forward to the outlet every week that makes you feel good.

KEY #2

TO HAVING AN ACTIVE MIND AND BODY IS KEEPING YOUR RELATIONSHIPS HEALTHY.

Why you ask? Because relationships take work. Working at something automatically kicks your brain into high gear.

I am going to break my relationships into five pieces. You may have different pieces, but for me they are my partner, friends, parents, siblings and children. They are not in any order of importance. For me, each must be healthy, in order for my life to feel complete and happy.

PARTNER

Let's start with your husband or partner relationship. An important step to keeping your relationship strong with your partner is scheduling couple time. And try not to let your couple time get stale by always doing the same thing. Make a list together of the things you both like to do and pick some various activities. Think back to when you were first dating. What did you like to do together? Of course the first thing that comes to mind is sex. Well, yes, sex is important. And it is usually a huge factor in keeping a relationship strong.

Now we've all heard of how intimacy affects men and women differently. That's OK. The super-important thing to remember is that it is part of a healthy relationship. There have been many studies to show this. Of course sex can become the same old boring thing, blah, blah, blah... So... spice it up. Send the children to sleepovers and make the house romantic. Fix a nice dinner, have a glass (or bottle) of wine and put on some nice jazzy, romantic music. Go to a store you'd find on Bourbon Street and surprise your husband with something 'spicy'. Believe me, you will both get a good laugh to say the least. And who knows, maybe it's the 'spice' for which you've been looking. Lastly and most importantly, leave the tv off. The tube can ruin a romantic night.

I'll share a slightly embarrassing story about a 'spicy' party to which I was invited a few years ago. There's a home business named Passion Parties and if you sign up for a party at your house you get a discount and free products for yourself depending on how much your guests spend. So one of my best friends invited me to her party she was hosting. Since I rarely get to see her, I thought it would be fun to spend time with her and get a good laugh at the same time, so I went. At a Passion Party you buy romantic items that you can use with or without your partner in the privacy of your bedroom. The saleslady passes each item around the circle of guests and describes (in detail!) each item.

So as we are drinking wine and laughing at these products, I decided I must be getting old because, one, I really wasn't embarrassed as we were inspecting each item's bells and whistles (literally some had bells and whistles), and two, none of the products even interested me.

So I bet you're wondering if I made a purchase anyway. Yes, I did, and I've regretted my $80 ripoff purchase ever since. So here's the embarrassing part of it... I came home one day to find the delivered box had been opened by one of my children. No words were ever spoken and to this day I have no idea which one has more birds-n-bees education than the other.

So my point here is that the REAL fun was drinking wine with one of my oldest and closest friends who I definitely enjoy and miss, and catching up with her. The secondary fun was laughing with my partner about my purchases. Friends rock and making an effort to keep in touch is worth every second. The party was worth it because I laughed a lot that night and I released some good endorphins. Wow, I guess with age comes wisdom, and finding that very few things are embarrassing anymore (unless your teenager is involved). Try to find humor in everything, it is uplifting and just plain fun.

FRIENDS

I want to talk more about girlfriends. Somewhere I read a statistic that states women talk TWICE as much as men. I don't have scientific evidence on this one, but based on my personal experiences, it is true. How in the world do we have so much to say and how can we say it all at the same time? It's the strangest phenomenon to hear a group of women talk and not know who is saying what, but knowing that they all hear every word of what everyone is saying. How is this possible? Some say it's the joy of women being able to multitask. Others say it's the rush we get when we all have to share what's going on in our lives with so little time to get it all out. I'm not really sure how we do it, but I know I like it, it works and I feel alive after a good girls' happy hour.

I remember the first time my partner, Stephen, met my family. My mom is very outgoing and from Savannah, GA so she has the Southern hospitality and enjoys conversation. My sister is also outgoing and enjoys a party. We had a gathering, like dinner at someone's house, and my mom, sister and I had our 'normal' conversation at the dinner table. Well, what we call 'normal', anyway.

After everyone left he had the most dumbfounded look on his face. He said, "How in the hell did you have any possible idea of who was saying what?" I just looked at him, just as dumbfounded, and asked "What?" "The three of you. You were all talking at once!" he said. "And...?" I said. "How could you have possibly understood the conversation?" he said. "I have no idea, but we did," I said. To this day, twelve years later, he is still amazed at our crazy way of conversing. Now he just shakes his head and turns to my dad, who is more his speed. They talk about guy things I guess, and both pause, a lot. The wine and beer help too.

So girls' weekends are one of the joys in life that all women should experience. I went to Randolph-Macon Woman's College so maybe for me it is like going back to school. My school was very small and intimate and it wasn't unusual to go to class in your pajamas. After all, there were no guys to impress and the professors certainly didn't care. Consequently every day and night WAS a girls' weekend.

So now a weekend away with my girlfriends brings back old memories and is one of the most uplifting and refreshing experiences ever. I have a group of friends from the last ten years from my children's school and their activities, and I have my college friends from 20+ years ago Last year six of us from college got together at my house for a weekend full of laughter, wine, chocolate and funny old photo album memories (GIANT hair from the '80s). This year we met in NYC and it was just as fun. If you haven't experienced a girls' weekend, you must. They truly are a blast.

If you find it challenging to get away for an entire weekend, then make plans locally for happy hours, movies, dinners, Bunko or anything that gets you away for a few hours and into an atmosphere of the crazy talking and laughter of women. You will leave feeling refreshed and ready to tackle your life again in the morning.

So let's recap a little. We are discussing Key Number 2 to keeping an Active Mind and Body, which is under Step Number 1 to feeling A.W.E.S.O.M.E. We've discussed keeping your relationships healthy with your partner and with your girlfriends. Let's talk about keeping your relationships healthy with your family – parents, siblings and children.

PARENTS

For me I have had it super easy to keep a good, healthy relationship with my parents because they are amazing. They have been married over 50 years (wow, that's crazy) and they have taught me good morals, great work ethic, and numerous life lessons. I'm fortunate to have them around still. They live very close to me for six months out of the year and then they are snowbirds in Florida for the other six months. It is always a hard adjustment when they leave for the winter. Having parents on whom you can rely is a true gift. I make every effort to see them as much as possible because the wisdom that they share is always amazing and uplifting. Not to mention the laughter. We've always laughed a lot as a family.

If you are not as lucky as I to have amazing parents, then try to find a mentor. Sometimes an aunt or uncle can fill the shoes of a parent. I have two first cousins who are like siblings to me because they lived with us. My parents have been their mentors over the years and consequently my cousins have done very well. I'm pretty sure if my parents hadn't been able to take them in, they would not be the happy, healthy adults they are today. And remember, your mentor doesn't have to be a family member. I have friends who have used parents of friends as their mentors. Close friends work just as well. Find a mentor of an older generation and you will have a place to turn in a time of need.

SIBLINGS

I have one sister who is three years older. Growing up we had the normal sibling rivalry. She let me tag along sometimes, but with three years difference we had different friends and interests for a long time. As we got older we started to do a lot more together. I would say when she was in college we decided that it was kind of fun to hang out. And then our lives paralleled for a while. We got married six months apart and became pregnant at the exact same time. And then...we both went into the hospital the same day to deliver our first child. My parents were not very happy because at the time she was living an hour away from me and we were in different hospitals. I couldn't deliver that day so I went home for two weeks, but she delivered a healthy baby boy. My son was born exactly two weeks later and our boys have been very close ever since. Our second babies were born three months apart.

I remember a girls' weekend we had together at Bethany Beach years ago. Six of us, including my sister, went away for the weekend and five of us still were nursing. We all hooked up our breast pumps a couple of times a day and pumped away. By the end of the weekend I'm pretty sure modesty had flown out the window as we all pumped in the living room and the freezer was full of breast milk. Yes, we did label it! I love telling that story because it still makes me smile.

Brothers and sisters offer trust and comfort. Having a support system around you is another key element in having a healthy relationship. We've had a lot of fun raising our children together. Our 'babies' are now in college!

CHILDREN

Speaking of 'babies', let's talk about our fabulous children for a while. Your relationship with your children is one more key to feeling happy. But how do you feel that love every single day when you swear someone has replaced your 'sweet babies' with aliens from hell?

Because after all, I couldn't have given birth to aliens, so how are they now living in my house?

The teenage years were both wonderful and horrible. Yes, I know that's a little contradictory, but that's really how it was. One day (or minute) when they are happy and there's no drama from who knows where, they are wonderful. We will laugh at the dinner table, watch a movie or play the Wii. Those moments actually do happen. And then...

Flash forward (maybe three minutes) and bam! There's no talking, no movement, no waking, basically no anything. Are you alive? I start to wonder how to stop the alien in them from completely taking over their mind and body. If I ask for help with a chore, there's a sigh at the beginning of a completely incoherent answer. So I repeat my request which, duh on my part, summons the exact same incoherent answer. Do I walk away and do it myself? It would be so much less stressful if I did. What kind of message is that sending? Why is my child acting like the living dead? Did I act this way? Am I a bad mother? How can all of these questions flash through my head at the exact same millisecond of time? I think I'm going nuts! Blah, blah, blah...

The relationship you have with your children is ever changing because they are ever changing and believe it or not, you are ever changing too. As they grow, so do you. So how do you grow together in a way that satisfies everyone? How do you keep your relationship with them respectful, authoritative and fun all at the same time? And why is it so important to MY happiness?

Let's start by saying, if I could answer all of those questions I would be a millionaire. The only expertise I have is spending the last 20+ years being a mom and seeing how my children compare to others their same age. And before you judge me for comparing my children to others, be honest, we ALL do it. To be fair, it's kind of the only way of knowing how your children ARE doing.

Parents wear blinders, pure and simple. Rip off the blinders and be honest. Do I have a good relationship with my children? If not, why not? How can I improve it? Am I lacking as a parent somewhere? Do my children need help in a certain area? Am I avoiding getting them the help they need? If so, why am I avoiding it? Am I pushing my child in a positive way or a negative way? Again, I will stress, be honest. It will pay off. Finding the answers to some of these difficult questions will help you have a fantastic relationship with your children for your whole life. The key is to never stop asking questions and consequently never stop looking for answers.

I find that as soon as things are going well, a curve ball is thrown in there just to keep me on my toes. Maybe this is life's way of snickering at us, saying, "You're not done yet. Here's a new one." I'm not really sure. But I do know that it keeps parenting exciting and also, many times, frustrating. As soon as you think "Wow, my children are A-OK," something new crops up!

Here's my quick synopsis of my life's curve balls with my children. Here are my beautiful, healthy children ages 3 and 5 and then, bam, my daughter at age 3 years 11 months is diagnosed with Type I diabetes. One year later, bam, both of my children are diagnosed with celiac. One year later, bam, their dad moves to California. Bam, bam bam…there is nothing in the books about these parenting curve balls. Help!

Flash forward to now. Through years of time and some therapy, somehow, and believe me I don't know how, they are pretty darn good kids. But I am pretty sure that my other four relationship pieces had a lot to do with it. The love and support from friends and family is a huge part of their success. So not only do healthy relationships matter to your happiness, they are also directly linked to your children.

Hopefully most of you do have a good relationship with your children, as I believe (most days) I do. But, if you don't, dig deep. Ask teachers, coaches, grandparents and friends. Don't be afraid to figure it out. None of us is perfect. But having a good relationship with your children is a huge part of YOUR happiness.

Remember, Keeping Your Relationships Healthy is Key #2 to Having an Active Mind and Body. Your five relationship pieces are partner, friends, parents, siblings and children.

So are you wondering what all of this has to do with reaching your healthy weight, gaining energy, and finding emotional freedom and balance? Isn't it just about counting calories and exercising? The short answer is yes, calories and exercise do matter. However, the longer answer is that the motivation to eat clean, exercise, work on your mind, only come when you have mastered the 7 Secrets and you have on your A.W.E.S.O.M.E.! Keep reading…

KEY #3

TO HAVING AN ACTIVE MIND AND BODY IS ENJOYING YOUR CHILDREN!

I know, this sounds easy, right? But for some reason we get so wrapped up in parenting and everyday life that we forget they're fun! Let's be honest, it is really hard to enjoy anything, let alone your fabulous children, when you are dog tired.

When they were younger I remember rushing from work at the end of the day to pick up my children from daycare, then rushing home to do dinner and dishes, and then bath and bed. I used to dread bath time. I need to clarify a little. It all has to do with my daughter's hair. She has a head of hair that people would pay thousands to have. It is thick, curly and blonde and it was down to her butt. Beautiful, right? Not if you're the one who has to brush through it at night. It used to take me an hour with an entire bottle of conditioner. At one point I was buying the gallon jugs of conditioner from Sally Beauty

Supply. We would lather her head, let it sit and then start ripping. Finally when she was around 9, I said cut it or you do it. She wouldn't cut it so she did it. Why, I ask, did I not demand that sooner?! Now she has a handle on it and all those years of tears are just a fond memory.

When I think about what age I've enjoyed the most, I have a hard time coming up with an answer. When they are little it's the sweet, loving time. It's OK to hug, hold hands and sleep in mom's bed. It's a closeness that every parent needs to enjoy and embrace. I'll say that again. You need to enjoy and embrace it. Why? Because it ENDS!

When their dad left for California they were 6 and 8. This started a very special time for the three of us. We went from a house with a mom and dad to suddenly a mom only. What effect does this have on a young child to go from seeing their dad all of the time, to hardly ever? Who knows, however it couldn't be good. Therefore, I knew in my heart that I needed to spend the next couple of years focusing on them and making sure they felt loved and important.

The first thing that happened, and I don't remember how it started, was they both started sleeping in my room every night. They would alternate between one on the floor next to me and one in the bed. I don't remember at the time if I analyzed this, but my gut told me it was OK. I'm pretty sure it was good for all three of us (and the dog – he now had a sleeping partner on the floor). This went on for a year or two and then my son decided he was ready to sleep in his room. Thank goodness, because the 'floor bed' was getting on my nerves. But my daughter decided to stay – until she was 11!

If you asked me two years ago where my daughter wanted to go to college, I would have said somewhere close so she can still sleep in my bed. She was 11 and I seriously thought I could rent her room because she slept with me every night. At times when I was super tired and I didn't want to be kicked all night, I would want her in her own bed. However, just as that thought was coming out of my mouth,

I said (many times out loud), "She won't want to sleep with me one day." Flash forward to the magical pre-teen age of 12, I was right. On her 12th birthday I noticed a dramatic transformation. This cute little daughter who was attached to me 24/7 all of a sudden wanted nothing to do with me – at all.

The point to this story…time passes fast so enjoy every moment, the good, the bad and the ugly. She kicked me for five years and now it all seems like a distant memory. Go with your gut and let your children feel your love and commitment to them. It will pay off in the end. You will end up with a wonderful relationship for life. And after all, that is Key #3 to Secret #1 of feeling A.W.E.S.O.M.E.!

What comes after love and commitment? Pure fun and laughter. Ride bikes, play games, have a Wii tournament, get out the board games, Go Fish, fart, burp…whatever is your pleasure, just do it. Laugh, move and enjoy your time together. Mine are now in college and I do miss them. Don't let a day pass that you don't have a positive encounter. And last but not least, always tell them you love them. No matter what.

KEY #4

TO HAVING AN ACTIVE MIND AND BODY IS PARTICIPATING AND VOLUNTEERING IN YOUR COMMUNITIES!

I have three communities. If you belong to a church or another group, you may have more. My communities are my neighborhood, my city and my children's schools.

My neighborhood was named Hunt Meadow and we had a lot of community events for our residents. We had Easter egg hunts, Fourth of July parades, Halloween parades, Santa on the fire truck,

Memorial Day and Labor Day pool parties and a midsummer crab feast. I used to do every single event when my children were young and consequently I ended up with some great friends. To this day one of my best friends, Michel, who now lives in California, was my neighbor who I met at the pool. Our children were best friends for many years and even though they don't see each other very often now, they can easily pick up from where they were years ago. It's amazing how a childhood friend can be a solid friend for life no matter how close you live physically. What a gift that is.

I remember when Michel lived in Hunt Meadow and because both of our husbands were out many nights due to their work schedules, we would do the 'grab what you have in your fridge and bring it over for dinner' dinners. We decided that this was a great way to, one, clear out the leftovers from the fridge and, two, laugh, a lot.

I'd like to share our famous nine-martini night with you. Michel and her husband, John, are from California, so after ten years on the East Coast, they decided to move home. One night we decided to have one of our 'clear out your fridge' dinners as a mini going away party. Off to Michel's I go with my children, then ages 7 and 9, and who knows what else – a chicken breast, a half of a potato and five pieces of broccoli – probably. That's OK, she was a stay-at-home mom most of the time and she liked to cook, so most dinners were better at her house anyway.

The children were off playing and she mixed us a nice refreshing martini, which was her specialty. We started to laugh and think about the last eight years together and well, let's just say she kept mixing. After the first couple, I think we had a few tears, from laughter and sadness, and then somewhere in the night we ended up in her hot tub. And yes, we had on bathing suits. There was a small problem with the bathing suit, however. I have a long body and she has a very short body, so her bathing suit was a tad on the small side for me. As we're out enjoying the night in her hot tub, her husband arrived home from work. He walked out to tell us he was home, talked to us for a while, told us the children were OK (we were worried), and casually mentioned to me that I needed to fix the top of my bathing suit. As we both looked down, we noticed that only one of my boobs was inside the suit! The other one was nicely hanging out on the outside enjoying the night. What a sight to see – two drunken women with a mom boob exposed. Needless to say, John drove us home that night. And yes, I only lived two blocks away. And no, that night was never repeated.

Getting involved with your neighbors and finding a few great friends from your neighborhood are other great relationship sources. Not only did I find a great friend for life, but my children did as well.

My second community was Annapolis City. Doing some volunteer work at your local homeless shelter or soup kitchen is a great way to give back to your community and to feel great about yourself. The saying "it feels better to give than to receive" is a very true statement. Volunteering your time is one of the best gifts that you can give yourself. Knowing that you are helping someone less fortunate than yourself is a wonderful feeling.

My third community was my children's schools. This is another great place to keep your mind and body active. Volunteering your time and finding new friends are both benefits to this community. Don't wait to get involved because after elementary school the opportunities drop off tremendously. The PTA is an option for middle and high school, but you don't have the intimacy of going into the classroom like you do during the elementary years. Taking in cupcakes for a birthday, going on field trips, Halloween parades, Thanksgiving parties and Christmas pageants are all part of the elementary years. Once they enter middle school, forget it. The last person they want around is mom!

KEY #5

TO HAVING AN ACTIVE MIND AND BODY IS JOINING A CLUB!

There are all sorts of clubs. Check out your local newspaper and you will see a page dedicated to clubs. There are clubs to bike, hike, ski, run, row, read, knit...the list goes on. Looking to meet a new partner? Join a dating club.

When I was finally ready to date after my divorce, I joined the dating club Match.com. It was fun to connect and share myself with others who were in the same place. I am a pretty blunt person, so I decided that if I was really serious about meeting someone, then I was going to be completely honest in my profile. I put the ages of my children, the fact that I was not only a single mom, but that my ex lived in California and that I would under no circumstance put up with a cheater. I was looking for an honest, family man who wanted a monogamous relationship. I enjoyed the site because you could 'date' and 'break up' all in a matter of minutes. I could tell 20 seconds into reading a profile if he was worth pursuing or not.

So finally one day I came across Scardy22. He was a single dad, soon retiring from the Coast Guard, where he was a commander, and his children lived with him full time. Full time, really? So did mine. Wow, this man may understand my daily mayhem. So flash forward twelve years and Stephen (Scardy22) and I are still together. Somehow through the melee of five children and no ex-spouses to cover some weekends, we have survived. Let me assure you we've had our crazy and tough moments, but somehow our lives together continue.

So get out there and join a club. It may take you one step closer to finding your A.W.E.S.O.M.E.!

KEY #6

TO HAVING AN ACTIVE MIND AND BODY IS COOKING!

So I know a lot of you just sighed and said really, I hate cooking. Well, so do I, so I'm going to share some simple, and I stress simple, ways to cook really healthy food. Put away the recipes and think easy.

Cooking at home is very important for finding your healthy weight and keeping it off. So if you are a big eat out person, start thinking about reforming.

The three main problems with restaurant food are fat, salt and portion sizes. In order for restaurants to stay in business their food has to be delicious and economical. So their motto is to load it up with (bad) fat and salt and serve plenty of it.

I'm not saying never eat out again. That would be horrible. But when you are trying to lose weight and figure out what a healthy weight human should be eating, then cooking at home for a while is the way to go.

One of my favorite exercises for my clients is when I ask them to keep a food journal. Journaling for as little as three days can be eye-opening. Usually I get, "I had no idea I was eating so much!" "When I used the nutritional label on the package for serving size, I realized MY serving size was TWICE theirs!" How many times have you measured your cereal? Do it one day and you will realize what a ½ cup really looks like.

When you cook at home you can easily monitor the fat, salt and portion sizes. Educating yourself on these three important food issues can be life-changing. The other benefit is figuring out that you CAN cook and you CAN do it in a way that's healthy, quick and easy. When I learned how to come home and whip up a totally healthy, fast meal it was awesome. Having your kitchen organized is important, and I will talk more about that later in the book.

There are so many elements to having an active mind and body. Who knew cooking would be one of them? Thinking and chopping will take you miles.

Here are some ideas that have served me well. I usually take Sundays to prepare for the week, so now I just add a little cooking time in there and voila – no cooking for the first half of the week. How marvelous.

Make enough of these to serve your family for 2-3 days:

1) **Quinoa** _ You can leave it plain or make it a veggie confetti. Dice your favorite veggies and throw them in. Take the super-easy route and use frozen veggies. My children like plain old peas and corn. Tip: Frozen veggies can have more vitamins than fresh.

2) **Salad** _ The darker the veggies the better and go for the rainbow – dark green, orange, red, yellow, purple, white. As long as the veggies are not full of liquid, like cut tomatoes, your salad will last up to three days in the fridge. Forget iceberg lettuce, that was so '80s.

3) **Soup** – I love soup. There are so many options here. Get out the crock pot and let it go. Traditional chili, veggie, veggie and bean, split pea, tomato...there are endless options. Soups are great as meals, appetizers or after school. They can also be a super-easy way to load up on lots of veggies and get in your vitamins.

4) **Italian Pasta Bake** – You don't need a recipe, just wing it. Start with a large oven-safe dish with a lid. Now think layers like lasagna. Dump jarred pasta sauce on the bottom, then some lentil pasta, then some chicken tenderloins, then more sauce...you get it. Add some high quality organic cheese if you want, and veggies. I usually top mine

with cut-up onions, mushrooms and peppers. You can also throw in a bag of frozen veggies. Easy, easy...no recipes.
5) **Mexican Rice Bake** – The same as the pasta bake but use salsa and torn corn (gluten free) tortillas. Keep the sour cream and cheese high quality and organic. Again, no recipe.

When you cook with whole foods the possibilities are endless. Buy the veggies and meats that your family likes and stick with them. There's no need to reinvent the wheel, just think lean protein, veggies and good plant fat. You will be so satisfied and healthy. There's no need to buy already done meals when cooking can be so easy. Fresh, fun and quick is the name of the game. Oh, and frozen. I love plain organic frozen veggies for soups and casseroles.

So there's my quick advice on cooking. I don't love to cook, but I do love whole, fresh and healthy food. Bon Appétit!

KEY #7

TO HAVING AN ACTIVE MIND AND BODY IS SAYING NO!

Yes, I mean no. I remember learning this when I was recently divorced and my ex moved to California. My first instinct was SUPER MOM, I can do it all. I'll show you who the best mom in town is. Well, that didn't last long. I quickly found myself out of steam.

When I think back I realize how crazy I was. There was not a free day or night that one of my children didn't have a sport or an activity. Why did I do that?...probably to make up for the fact that their dad was out of their lives. And to prove to myself that the three of us would be just fine without him.

Years ago I remember my son asked for guitar lessons. Music, really, I never thought my children would ever play an instrument. How could I say no to him? So I looked at the calendar and I realized we had one free night all week. Perfect, let's do it. That guitar lesson was the straw on the camel's back. Being out every single night of the week was enough to send me into the nuthouse. Luckily my son had a very boring and strange instructor so the lessons soon ended, and my sanity was nicely reinstated. And no, he never asked for lessons again, but oh well.

Learn to say NO if it is simply too much. He can learn the guitar anytime, and it certainly didn't have to be when he was 10. Your children will find their own path so don't make yourself crazy by trying to find it for them. Say no and feel good about it. You're super important too. Believe it or not, your children will respect you more. They will start to understand that you're not just a chauffeur, but a person with a life. Be proud and parent with confidence.

So now that you can say no, what now? Remember what we've talked about so far. Join a club, go out with girlfriends, work out, cook, volunteer, have a date with your husband... you know what to do, so get out there and do it.

THE SECOND SECRET TO FINDING YOUR A.W.E.S.O.M.E. IS EATING WHOLESOME FOODS!

Eating wholesome foods is very simple. Here are your categories:

1. Carbohydrates: vegetables, fruit, gluten free grains
2. Protein: plant, lean animal
3. Fats: plant
4. Sugar: natural and unprocessed
5. Condiments and Spices
6. Water

As you can see, plant is a big word here. The more plant-based your diet is, the healthier you will be. That's science, and my opinion. So let's get into more details.

FOOD #1

IN WHOLESOME FOODS IS VEGETABLES (OF COURSE!)

Vegetables, of course, you know it's all about the vegetables. I know you've heard it before, if you want to lose weight, then eat more vegetables. Well, I hate to break it to you, but it's true, and it's true for more than one reason.

The obvious reason is vegetables are low in calories and full of fiber. The second and more important reason is they are good for you. And I'm not saying this lightly, they are really good for you. Their vitamins, minerals, and antioxidants help prevent cancer and all sorts of other diseases.

Let's start with the low in calories. Your basic non-starchy veggies – lettuce, carrots, peppers, celery, broccoli, asparagus, mushrooms, onions…the list goes on – are basically what I call free foods. They are low in calories and barely affect your blood sugar. If you want, you can eat them all day and they won't make you gain weight. They may affect your digestive tract, but they won't give you extra pounds.

Most vegetables hold a lot of water and are good sources of insoluble fiber, meaning the fiber does not absorb water from your digestive tract. This is why large amounts of vegetables, like giant salads every day, will make you go to the bathroom, sometimes more than once a day. I like to call them "movers" if you will. They simply help everything move through your system. If you suffer from constipation, this is your first line of defense.

I tell all of my clients that you have to eat to lose. And I don't say this lightly. You have to eat a lot. How do you eat a lot and expect to lose weight? You eat a lot of low-calorie food like vegetables. But remember, this is just your appetizer. Think of giant salads and piles of vegetables, like broccoli, as the start to each meal. It's your first line of defense to feeling full. If you stuff yourself with vegetables before your protein and healthy carbs, you will eat less of the higher-calorie foods. If this sounds too simple, then think again. It's not. It's really this simple. Bulk up on vegetables before your meal. It's basic and simple and it works. If you are used to eating one serving of vegetables with a meal then make it four or five servings. Yes, that much. Add some lean protein, healthy plant fat, like avocado, and high-fiber nuts to your giant salad and make it your meal.

So even though your main goal is to get to your healthy weight, the other goal, which technically is more important, is to nourish your body. One hundred years ago there was no processed food. People ate from the ground. They literally ate from the ground, whole, real, nourishing foods that were full of vitamins, minerals, fiber and antioxidants. The only reason the life span was less was because doctors couldn't cure diseases and fight infections like they can today. That's the ONLY reason. I guarantee people were much healthier from the foods they ate.

Eat the rainbow. Eat your medicine. Think color and phytonutrients.

There's a reason vegetables are so colorful. They're beautiful because they want you to eat them. Their colors pack a punch of vitamins, minerals, and anti-inflammatory and antioxidant compounds that are called phytonutrients. White is the only exception to the color rule. Make sure you include whites like onion and garlic so you don't miss out on some very important nutrients.

Let's review what each color has to offer. I'll list vegetables and fruit together.

Red: tomatoes, pink grapefruit, watermelon

The color red signifies carotenoid lycopene, which is an antioxidant. It helps protect a person from getting cancer, especially prostate, and helps protect against certain diseases, like heart and lung. You actually get more lycopene from cooked tomatoes rather than raw, so eat that tomato sauce. Also, if you're a juice person, go for tomato juice. One glass gives you 50% of the recommended lycopene.

Yellow/Green: kale, spinach, collard greens, turnip greens, mustard greens, yellow corn, green peas, avocado, honeydew melon

These are loaded with lutein and zeaxanthin, which are carotenoids. Carotenoids are believed to help keep your eyes healthy. They help reduce the risk of cataracts and age-related macular degeneration.

Orange: winter squash, sweet potatoes, pumpkin, cantaloupes, mangos, carrots, apricots

These contain alpha carotene and beta carotene, which protect the body from cancer and help repair damaged skin. Beta carotene also is converted to Vitamin A.

Orange/Yellow: oranges, peaches, nectarines, tangerines, papayas

These contain beta cryptothanxin, which may help prevent heart disease. They are also high in Vitamin C.

Red/Purple: red wine (yea!), prunes, blueberries, red apples, strawberries, eggplant, beets, purple grapes, blackberries

Anthocyanins. These are the powerful antioxidants believed to prevent blood clots and thus protect against heart disease.

Green: kale, broccoli, Brussels sprouts

Kale – the number one superfood. I love, love kale. These are huge cancer fighters. They contain sulforaphane, isocyanate and indoles. They are believed to be the best cancer-fighting foods out there.

White / Green: garlic, onions, pears, white wine, chives, endive, scallions, leeks

Allicin is the compound found in the onion family that is thought to have tumor-fighting agents. Quercetin and kaempferol are also in this group and they are antioxidant flavonoids.

So there's the lowdown on your veggies. There's only one, very simple thing to remember about vegetables...they fight disease! If you want to live your life free of cancer, heart disease, liver disease, and the list goes on...then eat your veggies. And a lot of them!

Here are some ways to enjoy vegetables:

- Just eat them
- Cut up different varieties and stir fry in some olive oil and spices
- Mix them all together to make a giant salad
- Cut them up and serve with dip or hummus
- Blend in a smoothie – like kale
- Mix into soup and chili
- Puree and add to pasta sauce
- Puree to make a soup

You know what to do, so enjoy.

FOOD #2

IN WHOLESOME FOODS IS FRUIT!

I love fruit. It is the perfect snack when paired with some protein and fat, like nuts. It has vitamins, minerals, fiber and so much goodness that it's hard to list everything positive. Along with vegetables, fruits help fight disease and prevent cancer.

The number one complaint I hear about fruit is it has too much sugar. It doesn't have too much sugar; it has naturally occurring sugar and no added sugar. There is a vast difference between the two.

Fruit has its sugar born into its flesh. It ripens on the tree or bush and turns into a lovely, sweet piece of goodness. The fruit has a beautiful, protective skin that no human has touched, pierced or processed. It is natural and lovely. It is what we call a whole food.

Foods that have added sugar are called processed foods. They have been touched, pierced and prodded by humans. My favorite sugar example is the "healthy" fruit snack. All I can say about fruit snacks is, really? Is it really possible to have fruit and snack in the same phrase when all that's in this "healthy" kid snack is...sugar? Isn't that just a little deceiving? And it's not even good sugar from sugar cane or beets. It's usually high-fructose corn syrup, which is another man made substance. HFCS is made in a lab by injecting powerful chemicals into a corn stalk to extract its sugar. Really? How gross! And this is what we're giving our children? And then they add partially hydrogenated vegetable oil, which is a big artery clogger. Can you hear me ranting? It truly makes me crazy!

OK, so back to our fruit discussion. All-natural, lovely fruit makes me happy. Eat fruit, feel the goodness and enjoy its juicy loveliness. It's the healthiest carb out there. Go for 1-2 servings a day.

Here are some ways to enjoy fruit:

- Just eat it
- Cut up different varieties and make a fruit salad
- Mix it into your oatmeal
- Top it with natural nut butter
- Blend it into a smoothie
- Cut it up in cereal or yogurt

You know what to do, so enjoy.

FOOD #3

IN WHOLESOME FOODS ARE ORGANIC NON-GMO GRAINS!

Why do I specify non-gmo (genetically modified organisms) organic grains? Because genetically modified gluten containing grains are creating tons of health problems.

Gluten is a protein in wheat, rye, and barley. In the 1950's microbiologists genetically modified wheat, rye, and barley so that they would be resistant to the herbicide, glyphosate. Glyphosate is the organophosphorusin compound in the herbicide, Roundup. The herbicide is used in the fields to kill weeds and pests so that harvesting is made easier and the farmers yield 10 times more grain. And since the grains were genetically modified to resist Roundup, the grains are not destroyed. Normally Roundup would kill every grass in its path, but when a grass (grain) is genetically modified then it's not harmed.

So flash forward 70 years and scientists are now linking health problems to the 'new' gmo wheat, rye, and barley that our country eats. Gluten sensitivities, celiac disease, depression, obesity, diabetes, eczema, and many more health problems are linked to these 'new' gmo grains.

Does this mean that that YOU are sensitive to these gmo grains? Not necessarily. However I will say that most people are affected by them and don't know it!

Food sensitivities are tricky because symptoms can take up to three days to occur. If I eat gluten or dairy then I may have an eczema flare two to three days later. So if you've never done an elimination diet then you really will never know what foods may be causing your problems.

My friend Susan had psoriasis on her feet for ten years until she finally figured out through an elimination diet that gluten was causing her disease. Gluten had caused her feet to crack and bleed for ten years! When she went gluten free her psoriasis cleared 100%.

An elimination diet is not hard to do, but it does take patience. Typically people remove the top allergens from their diet until their symptoms improve, and then add each food back in one at a time.

Here's an example: Remove gluten, dairy, sugar, caffeine, alcohol, and eggs for two weeks. If your health improves then eat eggs for three weeks and monitor your health. If you stay healthy then eggs are not a problem for you. If eggs are a problem then remove them again and try another food. Keep a food diary so that you can keep everything straight. If none of the original foods clear your symptoms then you need to go deeper. Remove the next tier of foods like corn, soy, and nuts.

As you can see this is not a complicated process, but it is time consuming. Be diligent and you should come out of your elimination with some great data.

Here's my breakfast that I enjoy every morning.

Super Seed Oats with Berries and Nuts

Prep: Combine the following in a large container with lid

- 1 cup - organic gluten free rolled oats
- 1 cup - hemp hearts
- 1 cup - flaxseed meal
- 1 cup - coconut flakes
- 1 cup - cacao nibs
- 2 cups - chia seeds

⅓ - ½ cup of Super Seed mixture above

½ - 1 cup water OR Cashewgurt (Drinkable plain yogurt made out of cashews. Made by Forager.)

½ teaspoon cinnamon

¼ cup organic berries (frozen or fresh)

½ banana sliced (optional)

If you're using frozen berries then heat in the microwave for one minute prior to adding the banana. I prefer making the night before so the chia has time to swell, and then heating two minutes in the microwave in the morning.

A breakfast full of healthy carbs, protein, fiber, fat and antioxidants. This breakfast will keep you full for up to five hours. If your meal doesn't last you that long, then you need to eat more. The fat and protein are keys to satiety.

In addition to grains having protein, the other important ingredient that they offer is fiber. There are two kinds of fiber, insoluble and soluble. They are both important, but they function slightly differently in the body.

Some grains, like oats, have soluble fiber, whereas others, like wheat, have insoluble fiber.

Soluble fiber absorbs water. When you ingest soluble fiber, like in oats, it mixes with water in your digestive tract and forms a gel like substance. Your body works for a while to break down this gel substance and extract all of the good ingredients. This length of time that it takes your body to use fiber is what gives you lasting satiety. In other words, it makes you feel fuller longer. The key to not feeling hunger is giving your body foods that take awhile to break down. If they stay in your system for awhile then your hunger hormone is suppressed that much longer.

Insoluble fiber does not absorb water and mostly acts as bulk in your system to move everything through. Wheat and most non-starchy vegetables are examples of insoluble fiber. If you are a giant salad eater, like I am, you should notice your stools being slightly softer and your bowel movements being daily. A high volume of vegetables is the first defense against constipation. And if you eat too much, you will definitely know it. Back off a little and then build back up slowly over the next few weeks.

Many foods are a combination of soluble and insoluble fiber. One example is prunes. Prunes (or dried plums) have a tough outer skin that's insoluble, whereas the inside has a nice juicy pulp that is soluble. These are great for constipation. I love the no sugar and no preservatives dried prunes from Trader Joe's. They are also one of my favorites for a sweet fix. A couple of prunes always do the trick for me. Watch out, though, I ate too many one day, and regretted it the rest of the day.

To summarize grains, they offer protein and fiber, which are two very important components to satiety. The more protein, fat and fiber, the fuller you will feel and the longer you can go between meals. Lastly, and not to be overlooked, are the other nutrients you get from whole grains. They offer essential enzymes, iron, vitamin E and B-complex vitamins. Quinoa is my favorite gluten-free grain because it has a nutty flavor and it is has all nine essential amino acids, which is rare for a plant protein. Give them a try and I know you will be hooked.

FOOD #4

IN WHOLESOME FOODS IS PROTEIN!

Protein is an essential compound because it is needed for virtually every cell process in your body. If you eat animal products then it is pretty easy to get enough protein. But if you are a vegetarian or vegan, you do need to really concentrate on your daily protein intake.

You need between 33% and 50% of your body weight in grams of protein per day. I recommend going for 50% because then if you fall short it's not a big deal. So a 150-pound person needs around 75 grams of protein per day. If you don't think you are getting enough protein then keep a food journal for a day or two and add it up.

A good rule of thumb is to have protein every time you eat. This way you should achieve your daily grams of protein pretty easily, and protein keeps you satiated so you should feel fuller longer.

Protein is great for upping your metabolism, too. The harder your body has to work to break down a food, the higher the metabolic rate. The higher the metabolic rate, the more calories you burn. The more calories you burn, the more food you can eat. So eat protein at every meal and 'feel the burn'.

Fatigue and sugar cravings are two symptoms of too little protein. If you are feeling sluggish, up that protein.

Here are some good animal proteins:

- Fish (salmon, herring, sardines)
- Chicken breast (organic, free range)
- Turkey breast (organic, free range)
- Eggs

I don't recommend red meat or processed meats because research has shown that these meat eaters have a higher rate of colon and kidney cancer. If you do buy lunch meats, there are some available that are organic and preservative free. I buy Applegate brand, which is available at Whole Foods and Trader Joe's. They do not use nitrite, which is the preservative that researchers believe leads to cancer. Read your labels, and if there are too many ingredients don't buy it. You need to be able to pronounce the ingredients on the food label. If you feel like you're reading a foreign language, then leave it on the shelf.

Here are some good plant proteins:

- Organic Soy (a complete protein) – soybeans (edamame) and tofu
- Nuts and seeds (hemp is a complete protein)

- Whole grains (quinoa is a complete protein)
- Greens
- Beans and legumes

One of my favorite vegan recipes to keep on hand is a quinoa salad. This is a wonderful salad filled with tons of veggies, hearty plant protein and good fat.

Ingredients:

1 ½ cups quinoa

3 cups water

¼ cup lime juice

½ cup olive oil

1 cup kale, chopped with stems removed

½ cup carrots, chopped

½ cup scallion, chopped

½ cup green pepper, chopped

½ cup tomato, diced

1 can black beans, rinsed

Salt, pepper and other spices to taste

Soak, rinse and cook quinoa according to package directions. When cooking is complete, mix all other ingredients into quinoa. Add or delete ingredients according to what you have in your kitchen. Make enough to last a few days. Add an animal protein if you wish, or leave it vegan. Enjoy!

I didn't list dairy in the animal protein section because of how common it is to have intolerance to dairy. If you know for sure you are not lactose intolerant and you do not have any skin issues, like eczema, then use dairy for a protein source. I am dairy-free because I am lactose and casein intolerant and I have eczema. The lactose will give you painful gas and the protein, casein, will make you itch. Both of my problems have cleared up since going off dairy. It is a good protein source, but please evaluate yourself first before using. Believe me, the excess gas and itching are not worth it.

Don't forget your important protein. You need about 50% of your body weight per day. If you are craving sugar and feeling sluggish, keep a food journal and count your protein. You may be deficient.

Try your best to get most of your protein from plant sources. If you do eat animal protein, keep it lean. I cannot stress that enough. The leaner the protein, the better it is for your health. Red meat and processed lunch meats will clog your arteries over time and may lead to cancer. Leave them out of your diet. Salmon, herring and sardines have wonderful omega-3 oils so enjoy those in moderation.

Protein can be the forgotten food for women. We love our carbs! Eat protein with every meal and you should feel very satisfied.

FOOD #5

IN WHOLESOME FOODS IS SUGAR!

What, sugar is a wholesome food? Yes, because all food breaks down into sugar, even fat and protein eventually. Without sugar, our bodies would crash and burn. Sugar is our fuel.

There are two GOOD sugars and two BAD sugars.

1. Sugar that comes from organic sugar cane, organic honey, maple syrup and beets – GOOD!
2. Sugar that comes from whole foods – especially whole grains and fruit – GOOD!
3. High-fructose corn syrup that comes from corn stalks – BAD!
4. Sugar that comes from processed foods – white bread, white rice, granola bars – BAD!

Let's start with sugar number one – raw sugar from sugar cane, honey, maple syrup and beets. The best thing I can say about these sugars is – at least they're natural. A little bit in moderation, like sweetening your tea or coffee with them, is OK. It's much better than putting artificial sweeteners in your body that are made in a lab with chemicals.

One teaspoon of sugar has all of 16 calories and 4 carbs. Honey and maple syrup have around 30 calories per teaspoon and they pack some vitamins and minerals. Wouldn't you rather ingest a few calories with nutrients, rather than a ton of chemicals? The key to eating these sugars is moderation. I can't stress that enough. These are for slightly sweetening drinks and foods, but not living on them. Just a dab'll do ya because these sugars will spike your blood sugar and create internal inflammation.

Sugar number two is the important sugar. This sugar is made when our good foods, like whole grains, vegetables, and fruit, are broken down and digested. The importance of these sugars is that they slowly enter your bloodstream and gradually cause your blood sugar to rise. Keeping your blood sugar steady is the ultimate goal.

A steady blood sugar all day long will keep you satiated and will keep you healthy. If your blood sugar is not constantly spiking, then you will have good energy all day. You will avoid the 'peaks and valleys' of your blood sugar constantly going up and down. A steady blood sugar can help ward off diseases, especially Type II diabetes.

High-fructose corn syrup, the number three sugar, is a good example of a very bad sugar. Research now proves that HFCS creates high cholesterol and clogs arteries. There is nothing natural about how the corn syrup is extracted from the corn stalks. It is believed that high-powered chemicals and machinery are used which creates a toxic end product.

So why do manufacturers choose to use it? Because it's less expensive to produce high-fructose corn syrup than to grow sugar cane and beets. Money, money, money is of course more important than our health. It's such a shame and disappointment that our country allows such a thing. Stay away from all products with HFCS, they will spike your blood sugar, clog your arteries, and offer nothing healthy.

The last sugar is made from eating processed foods. Processed foods sugar and whole foods sugar are very different. When a food is processed, the manufacturer removes all of the good nutrients. Let's take the example of white bread. White bread started in the wheat field as a whole grain. But then someone decided it would make sense to remove the outer grain layers where all the nutrients live and come up with pretty, white, soft, squishy bread. Why? I have no idea. Marketing? Money? Taste? Probably.

So now that you have this pretty, squishy bread that children love, where are the nutrients that they need? Oh gosh, I'm sorry; we removed all of them to make you this pretty bread (product). OK, then put them back in. OK, we will. Here is your new enriched (fake) bread. You have all of the vitamins and minerals you need just by eating this pretty bread with fake nutrients. Did you say fake? Well, if they're not in there naturally, then I call it fake. The same goes for breakfast cereal and many other products. Enriching products because you fooled with their natural nutritious beauty, is well, in my opinion, stupid and criminal. Leave them alone and allow us to nourish our bodies with the wholesome goodness that is in our food. It seriously isn't rocket science!

Processed food sugar is another sugar that will spike your blood sugar. Since the food is already broken down, your body has nothing to digest. The sugar enters your bloodstream the minute you eat it. If there's no fiber or protein to digest, then your blood sugar rises immediately and you start on a rollercoaster of ups and downs. This is a very uncomfortable way to live. You feel highs and lows all day and those peaks and valleys can make it hard to concentrate, can give you headaches, and can give you severe fatigue. I don't know about you, but that is no way to live. And that is not how I want to spend my day.

If you want to know more about blood sugar then read up on glycemic index. The glycemic index of foods is the rate at which a food enters your bloodstream. It is quite interesting and can be a huge help for many people who need to eat a low glycemic diet because of Type 2 diabetes. The ultimate goal for Type 2's is to keep the blood sugar low and steady. A low glycemic diet will help you achieve this goal.

There's the quick lowdown on sugars. If you remember natural and whole foods you will be getting your sugar from all of the right places. Eat sparingly – raw sugar, honey, and maple syrup. Eat more frequently – fruit and organic non-gmo whole grains. This simple formula will make you feel amazing.

FOOD #6

IN WHOLESOME FOODS IS FAT!

Fat is wonderful. Without fat your brain would be mush, your arteries wouldn't run as smoothly, and you would be hungry all the time. Who wants that combo? I don't.

I remember in the '90s the diet craze was everything low fat or no fat. And I mean everything…'granola' bars, cereal, candy, and cookies. Of course I was a member of the highly processed, no fat, I'm going to look fabulous club. Who didn't want to be a member? Everything in the grocery was labeled Zero Fat. Great, I should be able to lose a ton of weight if I don't eat any fat. After all, if you eat fat then you'll be fat – right? Well, not so fast.

For some reason, one or two "studies" and one or two books about a new "diet" are enough to make the entire country jump on a bandwagon. This is what happened to me and so many others. I didn't lose weight on the No Fat Diet, but I sure did put a bunch of crap in my body and sent junk to my arteries.

Remember the oil Olestra? It was in foods like potato chips because it was an oil that your body could not absorb. So the flavor was in the food, but the fat was not absorbed in your body. No absorption equaled no calories equaled no weight gain. Wow, everyone was so excited that they could eat fat and not gain weight. Well, not really.

It did come with a warning that eating too much could give you gastrointestinal problems... diarrhea – that's lovely. Really – how disturbing. How gross is that; a food that's being ingested, but not being absorbed. Can there be anything more disgusting? Isn't food meant to nourish us? Aren't all the vitamins and minerals supposed to keep us healthy and lavish us in health? Then why, oh why, would such a product be developed and then actually sold to unknowing, stupid consumers, like me? Why would any government agency allow such a product to pass inspection? Politics, money, politics, money...you get the point.

The positive side to such a case is that I think, and I stress think, our nation is starting to wake up. Some authentic, scientific research is starting to take place and teach Americans about healthy eating.

The USDA changed from their outdated food pyramid to a new plate diagram. In my opinion it's only a slight improvement. In believe the plate should be ½ vegetables, ⅛ lean protein, ⅛ organic whole non-gmo grain, and ¼ plant fat. I don't think dairy should be included because it's a top allergen for most. The truth is, if you have a diet full of greens and fish, like kale and salmon, you can get your daily calcium from those foods.

So what fat should we eat? Plant, plant, plant, plant and more plant! Plant fat actually helps keep your arteries clear of plaque buildup, which can reduce your cholesterol. How cool is that? Concentrate on extra virgin olive oil, sesame seed oil, flaxseed oil, nuts, seeds and avocados. Keep in mind that this good fat is still calorie dense, so if you are watching your calories, be aware of serving sizes. Measure oils and nuts for awhile until you can 'eyeball' a serving.

As far as animal fat, eat it sparingly. I suggest poultry, eggs, and fish. I do not recommend red meat unless it is very lean, organic and grass-fed. And under no circumstance eat processed lunch meats that have preservatives in them. Research shows that processed meats are leading to colon cancer and possibly kidney cancer. Good quality, preservative-free meats are available at stores like Whole Foods and Trader Joe's. Organic Applegate lunch meats have no nitrates or nitrites, are antibiotic-free, are humanely raised, and are gluten and casein free.

Bison is one of the red meats that you can enjoy on occasion if you have to have your red meat. Buy it from a good butcher and make sure it's grass-fed. Grass-fed animals exhibit high levels of omega-3 fats because they are eating what they are meant to eat and they are able to roam free and exercise. This combination will give you a much higher quality of meat.

For poultry, keep it lean by eating the breast of the animal and not frying it. Fried chicken is an American favorite, but it is not the healthiest. Try oven frying instead. Dip the chicken in raw egg and then coat it with almond flour. Sprinkle your favorite herbs and spices on top and you now have a healthy 'fried' chicken.

Fish is one of my favorite foods. Three of my favorites are salmon, herring and sardines. I know most of you right now are thinking, yuck, herring and sardines! I know I used to say that too, but now I eat them on my salads and the benefits are wonderful. They pack a ton of protein, few calories, low to no mercury, calcium and wonderful omega-3 fats. For me, because the rest of my diet is vegan, I am able to get a good dose of protein and calcium for the day. Remember you need about ½ your bodyweight in protein each day.

Dairy is a good source of calcium and protein, and that is one reason the government keeps it on its food plate diagram. For some people who are not eating a balanced meal, milk provides calcium and protein. So if you are not sensitive to dairy, then at least you are getting those benefits from it. It's much better to see people drinking organic grass-fed milk than soda.

Some good organic grass-fed dairy products are full-fat cottage cheese, full-fat milk, and full-fat Greek yogurt, which has twice the protein of regular yogurt. Listen to your body. If you feel gassy after eating dairy and you suffer with eczema, eliminate it for a couple of weeks and see if your symptoms go away. You too may have an intolerance to dairy and not realize it.

Eggs have some fabulous health benefits. They contain antioxidants, choline, vitamins and minerals, just to name a few. However, because they are from an animal, they do have cholesterol. If your diet is primarily vegan, like mine, eggs can be a nice addition to your diet. One egg has 70 calories and 180 mg of cholesterol. I like to make a three egg omelet or scramble. Throw in some diced veggies and it makes for a great breakfast or dinner.

Remember fat is good as long as it is mostly plant, however, watch your serving sizes because fat is calorie-dense. Stock your kitchen with olive oil, nuts, avocados, olives, fish, boneless chicken breasts and eggs and you should be good to go. If you want to try vegan for a day go for meatless Monday. Physicians Committee for Responsible Medicine, PCRM.org, is a good vegan resource in case you are interested in learning more about a complete plant diet.

FOOD #6

IN WHOLESOME FOODS IS WATER!

Water is one of the most forgotten 'foods' out there. Drink water. Drink water. Drink water. Stop wasting your money on energy drinks and 'water with vitamins' – really? If you eat your vitamins and lose the sugar addiction, you won't need energy in your drink or vitamins in your water. Our bodies are hydrated with plain simple water. It's calorie-free and super-nourishing.

I've heard so many times, "I don't like the taste of water." There is no taste to water so how can you not like it? That's a strange one to me, but if that is the case with you, then add a little zest to it. Squeeze a lemon, lime or orange wedge and your water will take on a completely new life. It's truly amazing how far a citrus squeeze can go.

If you have well water with a lot of iron, then put it through a filter. The same goes for city water with the chlorine taste. Most refrigerators have water filters built right into them now. Mine makes the best-tasting water ever. There are also filters that attach to your kitchen faucet, whole house filters and pitchers with filters. You name it and it is probably made. Filter your water, hit it with a squeeze of fruit and you have a great beverage. If you are a serious athlete, add a touch of salt and sugar and you now have an all-natural sport drink with electrolytes. Serve your children this instead of the store-bought kind with artificial flavors and colors. Their bodies will thank you for it. If you want to make your own, here is a recipe. I tried it on my son and he loved it.

1/4 cup sugar or honey (choose your favorite)

1/4 teaspoon sea salt

1/2 cup hot water

1/4 cup 100% orange juice or apple juice or cranberry juice (choose your favorite)

2 tablespoons lemon juice or lime juice or a mixture of the two

3 cups cold water

Stir the sugar and salt into the hot water to dissolve and then add all of the other ingredients. Add less sugar if you want it more on the tart side.

Here's to a nice healthy sports drink. No artificial colors or ingredients and it's less expensive than the store-bought brands.

Another reason water is important is because dehydration can mimic hunger. Yes, dehydration can mimic hunger. Many times I have felt hungry only to realize I was really thirsty. Always go for a glass of water when you start to feel hunger coming on. It may save you some serious calories.

If you are still hungry after downing a glass of water, then it is probably time for you to eat. The good news is, since you have a full glass of water in your stomach, you will probably consume less food. Less food equals fewer calories. Nice! Keep that water rule in mind and you will save yourself from eating unnecessarily. Eat when you are hungry, but make sure you actually are hungry first.

Keeping hydrated with water will keep your skin healthy as well. Fewer wrinkles will show if your skin is plump and hydrated. Who doesn't want a free face lift.

Hydration keeps your kidneys and other organs happy, too. Drinking too little will lead to stagnant urine in your bladder, which can lead to a bladder infection. A bladder infection not caught in time can lead to a kidney infection, which can be very serious. Drink plenty of water to keep that pee running clear and the bacteria will flush out of your system.

Other areas affected by too little water are your circulatory system, your digestive system, and your brain. These systems don't function optimally when too little water is present. Your blood and digestion will move slower and your brain will start to feel achy. When I start to feel a headache coming on, many times I just need to hydrate. The body is amazing at telling you what it needs. If you do a good job of listening to your body, and not ignoring it, you will be amazed at what it tells you. As simple as your head not feeling right, may be the first sign that you need to drink. That's pretty amazing. Listening to your body will keep you healthy and alert. Ignoring signs and symptoms will take you down the sick path. Listen, listen, listen…

The last advice for staying hydrated with water is that it is a neutral drink. A neutral drink offers no calories and no addiction path. I'll say that again. Water, a neutral drink, offers no calories and no addiction path. These facts are extremely important for finding your healthy weight and living your dream-life.

Calorie-free is key for losing weight, because now all of your calories can go to food. I don't know about you, but the more I can eat the better. Put your calories toward food – it is a no-brainer.

No addiction path refers to diet drinks. Diet drinks are artificially sweetened, therefore they have no calories, but the artificial sweetness still tricks the brain into thinking you are eating. Don't miss this key point. The brain is tricked into thinking you are eating. Tricked, tricked, tricked. The brain thinks sweet, which means sugar or food, right? Well, no, not when the sweetness is artificial and offering no calories.

When the brain perceives food coming in, the body releases insulin to cover that food. Insulin is the hormone that transports the sugar from your food into your body's cells for energy. It removes the sugar from your bloodstream, sends it into your organs, and now you have energy to go about your day. So, if your body has no actual food coming in, then your blood sugar drops 'accidentally', sugar is removed from your bloodstream, and now you feel...hungry! Yes, you feel hungry. The brain cannot decipher between real sugar and fake, so it sends the exact same message to your pancreas, which is to release insulin. Voila – low blood sugar! Can you see how diet drinks are messing with you? They play tricks on you and actually increase your hunger. They increase your hunger. This is the wrong. Decreasing hunger is the ultimate goal. No more diet drinks, no more diet drinks, no more diet drinks. They play with your head, literally.

The other way artificial sweeteners negatively affect you is that your brain 'tastes' the sugar and wants more. Sugar is a drug. Yes, sugar or perceived sugar is actually a drug. There have been numerous studies to show that sugar affects the brain's hormones the exact same way as illegal drugs do. I know that sounds crazy, but it's true. Sugar is a drug. The more you eat, the more you crave. So even though you are eating 'fake calorie-free' sugar, your brain still thinks sugar, releases dopamine, the 'do it again' hormone, and now you want more sugar. This is an addiction. Sugar addiction is a very real problem and diet sodas are a main culprit. Staying away from diet drinks should help you crave fewer sweets. Craving fewer sweets should help you eat less. Eating less should help you lose weight. It's pretty cool to see how all of the pieces fit together in your 'health puzzle'. Wow, all of this just from drinking water? Water is the name of the game.

FOOD #7

IN WHOLESOME FOODS IS CONDIMENTS AND SPICES!

Condiments and spices are lifesaving – literally! Spices like turmeric and cinnamon are known for their anti-inflammatory and antioxidant properties. But I really can't single out those two because all spices are extremely good for you. Yes, every single spice is an excellent addition to any meal for the health benefits and for their taste. They all have unbelievable flavors that can dramatically change a meal.

The most common avenues for taste are fat, sugar and salt. Condiments and spices can help you get away from that path and put you on a much healthier and tastier path to eating. Instead of reaching for the salt, reach for cumin, oregano or parsley. Or maybe turmeric, sage, cinnamon and cloves are more up your alley. Pick some of your favorite spices and experiment. Cinnamon in chili is one of my favorite additions. Don't be afraid to try different combinations. Spices can be fun. First decide if you like a spice, and then try it out the next time you cook. It's that easy. The only way to start using spices is to just start.

Condiments can save a boring meal too. Sometimes plain baked chicken can be saved with ketchup, mustard, honey mustard, barbecue sauce, teriyaki sauce, sweet and sour sauce, cocktail sauce – you get the point. Keep a good array of condiments in your fridge and you can save any meal. A lot of people like simple because they like their own flavors. My son's two favorites are ketchup and honey mustard. I have a stack of the very small clear glass bowls and he uses two of those, one for each of his condiments.

Condiments have health benefits, too, as long as you check the ingredient list. Tomatoes in ketchup and the mustard seed in mustard are both antioxidants and good for you. I buy organic versions from Trader Joe's so there is no high-fructose corn syrup or preservatives in them. Healthy can easily be undone when adding HFCS to something. Always read the ingredient list to make sure your condiment truly is healthy. Some like barbeque sauce can have quite a bit of added sugar. Use those sparingly, but otherwise, pour on the ketchup or mustard and feel the healthy goodness.

As your body responds to these wonderful, whole foods you will quickly be on your way to finding your healthy weight. Read on for the exercise segment and start planning your AWESOME dreamlife now!

THE THIRD SECRET TO FINDING YOUR A.W.E.S.O.M.E. IS EXERCISING!

Exercise has so many benefits it's hard to list all of them. There are eight main benefits that keep me motivated. They are heart health, bone health, calorie health, sugar health, friend/partner/ you time, brain health, and example setting. Let's break down each benefit.

BENEFIT #1

IN EXERCISE IS HEART HEALTH!

In order to keep your ticker healthy you have to move. You can't do much with a sick heart, so move it or lose it. Exercising on a regular basis will keep your heart muscle strong, lower your blood pressure, and help keep your bones solid.

The American Heart Association recommends 150 minutes of aerobic exercise per week. That means three days a week for 50 minutes, five days a week for 30 minutes or seven days a week for 22 minutes. Whatever fits your schedule is what's best for you. I personally like five days a week and then if I fit in a fun exercise on another day, like biking or hiking, then it's just a bonus.

There's been a lot of research lately on interval training. The research suggests that interval training is an awesome way to go. You can easily add some to your daily walks. Pick a spot down the street, like a stop sign, and run as fast as you can to that sign. It should take you between 30 and 50 seconds to get there. Recover once you reach your destination for 10 seconds of regular walking and then resume your normal to fast pace. Do this four to five times during your walk and you will not only burn more calories, but you will also up your fitness level. It makes for an amazing workout. Give it a try, it is something achievable by all.

Heart-healthy food after exercise is important too. Eat a meal within 30 minutes after exercising so you don't become ravished with hunger and want to eat your own arm. Nice recovery food is fruit and nuts. Sticking to plant foods as much as possible will keep your heart healthy, too. The good fats in plants actually help reduce cholesterol.

It's pretty easy to keep that heart muscle strong, just move it and feed it plant food. It doesn't demand much.

BENEFIT #2

IN EXERCISE IS BONE HEALTH!

Bone health is becoming more of a hot topic than ever. Good bones need weight-bearing activity and calcium-rich foods.

Weightlifting is great for your bones if you don't like to do weight-bearing aerobic exercise, like running. Two 30-minutes sessions a week should give you some nice results. Of course, doubling that will make you look like a bodybuilder – ha, ha, I wish. As hard as

I work I still have a little chicken wing action on my triceps. I guess I'll just have to live with it, cluck, cluck.

Calcium-rich foods are also important for bone health. Milk and yogurt are on the top of the list, however, there are other foods with more calcium in them if you are not a dairy person. Don't fall into the trap of thinking you have to have dairy for your daily calcium. You don't.

Some great calcium-rich foods are:

- Kale, mustard greens, spinach, broccoli
- Sardines, salmon with bones
- Soybeans
- Almonds, sesame seeds
- Figs (I buy them dried at Trader Joe's and they are the best snack)

Ward off osteoporosis with some weight-bearing activity and some calcium-rich foods. It may be enough to keep your bones strong and healthy for life. Remember Popeye – eat that spinach.

BENEFIT #3

IN EXERCISE IS CALORIE HEALTH!

Calorie health is quick, simple and to the point – the more you move the more you burn. The more you move the more you burn. The more you move the more you burn. Blah, blah, blah...we've all heard it a gazillion times, but it's true.

The more you exercise the more calories you burn and consequently the more you can eat. Plain and simple – move so you can eat and keep that heart healthy.

There are a couple of ways to burn calories. Aerobic exercise burns most of your calories immediately while you're exercising and has a small after-burn. Weightlifting burns calories while you're lifting and has a large after-burn for up to 24 hours. All of this after-burn is what helps your metabolism stay high. If your body is looking for energy, it's going to let you know. What a great way to burn up that food.

BENEFIT #4

IN EXERCISE IS SUGAR HEALTH!

Exercise helps your blood sugar stay stable. OK, but what is blood sugar and why do I want it to be stable?

I learned way too much about blood sugar in 2002 when my daughter was diagnosed with Type I diabetes. In one day I was on blood sugar overload. Here's the lowdown.

All food is broken down into sugar. Carbohydrates are the fastest, followed by fat and then protein. When we eat, our body turns the food into sugar and deposits the sugar in our blood. Our brain now senses the sugar in our blood has started to rise (it needs to stay a certain level) and tells our pancreas to release the hormone insulin.

What is insulin and why do we need it? The hormone insulin is a transporter. It has one tiny, but very important feature, which is to transport the sugar from our bloodstream into the different cells of our body for energy. You wouldn't think this one tiny hormone would have such a dramatic effect on our body, but it's huge. If you don't have enough insulin to move the sugar out of your bloodstream and into your cells for energy, then you have no energy. If you don't have any energy then you will have severe fatigue and your body will not be able to operate properly.

Let me explain how Type 1 diabetes works because it is much easier to understand than Type 2 diabetes.

Type 1 diabetes is an autoimmune disease. For some reason the body kills off good cells in the body because it gets confused and thinks they are bad cells, like a virus. The immune system basically has a brain fart and goes haywire on good systems. This is what happened to Julia. Her immune system killed all of the beta cells in her pancreas that normally produce insulin. She was left with none. Consequently, she wears her pancreas now in the form of an insulin pump. When she eats she tells the pump how much insulin to give to cover her food.

The body likes a blood sugar in the 70-110 mg/dl range. This is where the body performs optimally. When Julia was diagnosed her blood sugar was around 450 mg/dl. She was extremely thirsty and she had become very thin. Because her body had no sugar to use for energy, it started to eat fat and muscle. This is called diabetic ketoacidosis and it is very dangerous. Death will occur if insulin is not administered in a timely manner. Luckily, she was alert and happy when diagnosed because I caught her diabetes early. Many children present in a coma because the diagnosis is missed and their blood sugar rises to over 1000.

So how does this relate to exercise and blood sugar? Exercise lowers blood sugar, which means you need less insulin to be released from your pancreas. In her case she needs to physically give herself less from her pump, but in a normal person the body needs to release less from the pancreas. OK, so why is this important? Research now shows that if you can preserve your insulin, then you may be able to stop blood sugar diseases from affecting you. If Type 2 diabetes runs in your family, then this means you. Type 2 diabetes has a strong family inheritance. If you know you could be affected one day, start now to preserve your insulin. Exercise could be your ticket to no diabetes. And if you already have diabetes, exercise will dramatically improve your control. Better blood sugar control equals happy and healthy organs – especially the heart and pancreas.

BENEFIT #5

IN EXERCISE IS FRIEND / PARTNER / ME TIME!

Exercise with friends, your partner or alone and work on those healthy relationships that are so important to having an active mind and body. If you're exercising alone, remember that having a healthy relationship with yourself is the ultimate goal in all of this. THE ULTIMATE GOAL! If having some alone time is good for you and you like to have it while exercising, then go for it. Make that time for you.

If on the other hand you need some motivation, seek out a friend or your partner for some heart-healthy workouts. You can motivate each other to stay regular with your workouts and you can talk and laugh together all at the same time.

Of course laughter can come at the expense of others, but that's just part of it. My friend does a lot of yoga and she is constantly busting up during class when the silence is broken by a giant fart. Farts are funny to me, so I know I would bust a gut. If you're not into farting, then stay out of the yoga room because I hear it is a common occurrence. And I don't know why farts are funny since we all do them. You would think we are all so used to hearing them that you could just fart anywhere and it would be accepted...well, not so much.

When you have made plans with someone to exercise, that is another great motivator. It is pretty easy to back out on yourself, but not as much when someone is counting on you. There are many people who exercise regularly just because they have a workout buddy. This is totally OK. If you need it and it works for you then go for it.

One of the things that saved me during my divorce was my morning neighborhood walks with my girlfriends. We met most mornings after the children were in school and just walked and talked. All of those talks saved my life. I truly believe that. We hashed out everything that was going on with me, got our Vitamin D from being outside and received our serotonin boost. Those mornings helped me heal many times faster than I would have if I had stayed a hermit in my house.

So exercise with a friend, partner or yourself. Whatever works best for you is what's best. Get out there and move. Feel the burn and smile a lot.

BENEFIT #6

IN EXERCISE IS BRAIN HEALTH!

When I think about brain health I have a smile on my face and I feel happy eyes. Whenever a mouth smiles, the eyes smile, too. Do you know what I mean?

Why do I say this in reference to brain health? Brain health equals a happy mind on the inside with a happy face on the outside. Sometimes you can alter the inside by smiling on the outside. If I feel grumpy I can smile and feel better. I know I look like an idiot, but it really can work. When you're in stopped rush hour traffic the next time, and you have on a frown face, just smile. You may be amazed. I usually end up smiling for real because I feel so stupid fake smiling. Give the silliness a try. After all, there's nothing else to do.

Have you ever smiled subconsciously? Apparently when I watch my funny shows at night I don't laugh out loud, but I sit quietly and I have on a perma-smile. I never knew this until Stephen pointed it out one night. I think I do this in funny movies, too. Maybe I'm not a laugh-out-loud kind of person, but I'm a quiet smiler. Either way, smiling or laughing are both super-healthy because serotonin is released with both. And remember, serotonin is our natural antidepressant. So when you're faced with the option of a crime scene show or a sitcom, go with the sitcom every time. You will feel much fresher at the end than if you watched a scary murder mystery.

So how does all of this tie into exercise? Exercise is the precursor to smiling. When you exercise you produce serotonin, the natural antidepressant, then you smile and now you feel even better. You now have a double dose of serotonin – some from the exercise and some from smiling. It's crazy how all of this works together. Don't you love the human body?

Exercise, smile, exercise, smile...just keep doing it and you will have amazing brain health and happiness for many years.

Lastly, exercise promotes brain health because it is an achievable goal. We all need life goals and taking a walk every day or pumping some iron a few times a week is super-easy and achievable. Feeling overwhelmed in life is very common. If you can take small, tiny steps toward a goal and achieve it, your life can feel much more manageable. If this sounds too easy, it's not. It's really that easy. Taking small bites out of your daily schedule can make the rest of your day move more smoothly. We all can exercise. It is possible. Make it a goal and just do it. Your now healthy brain, along with the rest of your body, will thank you for life.

BENEFIT #7

IN EXERCISE IS EXAMPLE SETTING!

This one is so important...exercise so your children will too. When you do something, your children usually emulate you. So the more you exercise, the more they will. It's a super-easy way to pass along fitness to your children and to hope that they will keep up the good habit for life. If they see you eating bags of chips on the couch every day, then they will sit down and join you. If, on the other hand, they see you riding your bike every day, chances are they are going to hop on their bike and join you. Setting good examples is part of the parent handbook. Make exercise one of them.

Let's recap a little. We're talking about the seven secrets to feeling A.W.E.S.O.M.E. and we have now finished Secret A, Secret W and Secret E.

SECRET A = ACTIVE MIND AND BODY

Key #1 is keeping your brain alive. Spice up your life by putting some fun stuff on your calendar. Do this for you, you + partner and family.

Key #2 is keeping your relationships healthy. My five relationship pieces are my partner, my parents, my sibling, my friends and my parents. If there's a conflict, work it out.

Key #3 is enjoying your children. Along with parenting, have fun with them! Laugh, ride bikes, play games – whatever is your pleasure.

Key #4 is getting involved in your community. You can get involved in your neighborhood, your city or your children's school. It makes you feel good to give back for free.

Key #5 is joining a club. There are so many out there, just pick your favorite. Knit, run, read…

Key #6 is cooking. Oh the joy of cooking. Cook some bulk items on Sunday and think simple. No recipes needed.

Key #7 is saying NO. That's right, just say no. If you are overbooked and cranky then turn something down. It's OK and it will keep you sane.

SECRET W = WHOLESOME FOODS

Food #1 is vegetables. Eat a rainbow of vegetables and a lot of them. They are high in antioxidants, high in fiber and low in calories.

Food #2 is fruit. Eat a rainbow of fruit. Fruit is high in antioxidants, high in fiber and a good carbohydrate. If you are looking for something sweet, fruit is your go-to food.

Food #3 is grains. Whole grains like quinoa are important for their protein and fiber. They will keep you satiated and give you a nice slow-burning carb for energy all day.

Food #4 is protein. Protein is important for your body to function properly all day. You need about ½ your body weight per day and protein ups your metabolism.

Food #5 is sugar. Sugar in fruit is healthy and good. Added sugar like in soda and processed foods will add calories but no nutrients. It is also very addictive!

Food #6 is fat. Most of your fat should come from plants. Second to plant fat is lean poultry, fish and eggs. Fat helps with satiety, but watch your portions because it is calorie-dense.

Food #7 is water. Water is important because it keeps you hydrated and allows your body to perform optimally. Switching to water from diet drinks also can help you get rid of a sugar addiction. Drink up before eating, because thirst mimics hunger.

Food #8 is condiments and spices. Condiments and spices are a great way to improve your health because they are loaded with antioxidants. You also can turn a boring meal into a lively meal just with a few additions from your spice rack or fridge.

SECRET E = EXERCISE

Benefit #1 is heart health. Aerobic exercise helps keep your heart muscle strong and helps lower your blood pressure. 150 minutes per week is recommended.

Benefit #2 is bone health. Weight-bearing exercises, like lifting weights, help keep your bones strong and your balance on track. Eat calcium-rich foods like kale and sardines to help ward off osteoporosis.

Benefit #3 is calorie health. The more you exercise, the more calories you burn. The more calories you burn, the more food you can eat.

Benefit #4 is sugar health. Exercise lowers your blood sugar, which means you need less insulin. Using less insulin helps preserve your pancreas and may help delay blood sugar diseases such as Type 2 diabetes.

Benefit #5 is friend, partner or me time. Motivation and laughter from a friend or partner during exercise will help keep you going on a regular basis. If you need alone time, then exercise by yourself.

Benefit #6 is brain health. Serotonin is the key to a happy brain. Exercise makes us happy, which makes us smile, which releases serotonin. This natural antidepressant keeps our brain healthy.

Benefit #7 is example setting. Your children will exercise and eat healthy if they see you doing it.

There are four more secrets to go…

S = Sleep

O = Organization

M = Mindfulness

E = Envisioning and Living Your Life True Life

THE FOURTH SECRET TO FINDING YOUR A.W.E.S.O.M.E. IS SLEEPING!

Seriously, all you have to do is sleep. It's that easy. I bet you're smiling from ear to ear now because you know this is the easiest secret in the book, right? Yes, it really is so simple; however, you still have to do it. Do NOT compromise on your sleep. The research suggests that sleeping between seven and nine hours a night is ideal. I usually wake up after 7.5 hours so I know that's my magic number. Experiment on the weekend by timing yourself and not using an alarm clock. You will be able to figure out how many hours is right for you.

If you are sleeping enough hours but you are not feeling rested, it may be for a few reasons. The first and most common reason is caffeine. Caffeine, or stimulants in general, can cause insomnia because the brain's sleep cycle is not allowed to perform properly. Coffee, tea, diet pills and decongestants are some examples that may be keeping you up at night. Try not to take any stimulant after noon. Some reports say caffeine can stay in your body for up to 10 hours.

Alcohol also can cause sleep disturbances. Alcohol is a depressant and should help put you to sleep, however, it actually can act in the opposite way. Alcohol can disrupt your sleep cycle. There are five stages to sleep:

- Stages 1 and 2 are light sleep
- REM is where you dream and it is considered light sleep with rapid eye movement
- Stages 4 and 5 are deep sleep

Alcohol robs us of stages 4, 5 and REM, thus leaving us in the light 1 and 2 stages. This is why you can feel very restless during the night after drinking alcohol before bed. Some people are more sensitive than others. I can be fine with one glass of wine, but two can make me wake up all night. During college I just used the 'pass out' method (ha ha), which seemed to work very well back then.

Keeping your room cool is also essential to a good night's sleep. Your body temperature rises during the night, so keeping your room cool and being able to control your heat with the covers will be more conducive to staying asleep. I have an automatic control on my thermostat that will change the temperature at different times of the day. During the winter I keep my house at 68 during the day and 64 at night. Experiment and see what temperature works for you.

Circadian rhythm is the last piece of the puzzle. We all have a natural 24-hour cycle. If you can go to bed and wake up at the same time every day you will keep your natural rhythm in harmony. If you can't, then sleep disturbances may be common. People who work night shifts can easily feel tired and out of sorts all of the time.

Keeping a journal can help you figure out what is waking you up in the middle of the night. Write down food, exercise, drinks, medicine, bedtime, wake time and supplements. The more information you write down, the easier it will be to figure out what may be hindering your sleep. If you can figure it out and you end up getting a great seven to nine hours then you should feel amazing every day.

If, on the other hand, you're not getting enough sleep because you don't think it's important, then read on to see what you're missing. It's extremely important and I lecture my children all the time about not sleeping enough. Get your sleep!

BENEFIT #1

FOR SLEEPING IS A SUPERCHARGED IMMUNE SYSTEM!

Who doesn't want a supercharged immune system? I do not like being sick, ever. Sleeping enough will allow your body to repair itself and send out attack signals when necessary. If your body doesn't have to fix itself from lack of sleep, then it can more easily attack any foreign invaders that may come its way. Your immune system will be at the top of its game with enough sleep.

When my children were young, I was sick all of the time. It may have been a combination of them bringing home viruses and me being run down from lack of sleep, but all I know is that I was constantly hacking up a lung. I had colds on top of colds.

The body is an amazing piece of machinery. It knows exactly what to do and when, as long as its owner provides it with what it needs. Sleep is the absolute easiest way to nourish your body. Remembering that too little will cause a ripple effect of bad things to come, should help you want to slumber more. Cozy up, climb in and enjoy those eight hours. You deserve it after a long day and your immune system will thank you for it.

BENEFIT #2

FOR SLEEPING IS GROWING!

Yes, this one's for your children. Getting the right amount of sleep starts as an infant and continues into adulthood. Infants need around 16 hours a day, children 10-12, teens nine and adults seven to nine. This is particularly important the first 18 years of your life because this is when you grow. Growth hormone is released while you sleep so if you're not sleeping enough, then it's possible that you're not growing to your full potential. I'm not going to get into too much science, let's just say that it makes sense to sleep enough so your hormones are given a chance to perform optimally.

Teens have it hard. Just as puberty is kicking in and their hormones are going wild, they have a huge load of school work and activities to balance. Aside from hormones, the circadian rhythm of teens turns upside down. They turn into scary night creatures wanting to stay up super late and sleep until noon. My son made Xbox LIVE dates with his friends on the weekend that started at 11 p.m. and ended somewhere around 3 a.m. He usually appeared at noon the next day. This worked for the weekend, but once the week started he was like the walking dead. And all of my efforts to get him out of the pattern failed.

One thing he did do was take naps. I wish he would have just pushed through and gone to bed early, but no such luck. He crashed on the couch every day and then he was wide awake again at night. I guess some things never change because I remember doing the exact same thing when I was his age. It's just something teens have to work through. After all, one day they will be rising and shining with the rest of the world and hitting that office.

The good news is that as long as the sleep debt is not too severe they do grow. My son is now 6' 3", so his funky sleep / nap schedule must have worked fairly well.

BENEFIT #3

FOR SLEEPING IS BRAIN HEALTH!

Clear thinking is what I strive for everyday. Who doesn't want to feel at the top of their game every day? Vibrant, quick thoughts help you achieve your daily goals in the most efficient manner possible.

I don't know about you, but I can definitely notice a change in my memory as I get older. Things that would have stuck in my brain easily 20 years ago, seem not to stick so well anymore. I have to concentrate a little bit harder and live by my online calendar to keep it all together. I call it selective memory because I give myself permission to remember what I want to remember and dump all of the junk. Ah, the beauty of getting older.

So how does this relate to sleep? Getting enough sleep will enhance your memory. As your body sleeps, it regenerates many systems and one of them is in the brain. The more our brain is allowed to recharge through the night, the better our memory will be the next day. The rest will organize and archive memories. If memories are organized and archived then they will be available for use.

Have you ever thought about how your brain feels the day after a sleep-deprived night? We all recognize that we feel tired and sleepy, but how many think about cognitive thought? I feel fuzzy brained. I want to recall certain things, but my brain doesn't want to cooperate. My memory feels tired and unavailable. This is all due to sleep debt.

I don't know about you, but now that I'm in my fourth decade of life I need all the help I can get in the memory field. I love my solid 7.5 - 8 hours of sleep every night and I will fight to my death to get it. Give me nine on the weekend nights and I'm good to go for the next week. Wake me only for fire or profuse bleeding. Other than that, enter at your own risk.

BENEFIT #4

FOR SLEEPING IS BEAUTY SLEEP!

Need I say more? It's true, the more you sleep the better you look. Dark, yucky circles are so hot and I know we all love them, right? Well, you can easily have them by not sleeping. However, if you want bright, vibrant eyes that look clear and crisp, then get your eight hours.

When we sleep the recommended amount, our body has sufficient time to repair itself. This includes muscle, tissue and cells at every level. Visible signs that our body is not repairing itself sufficiently can include stringy hair, wrinkled skin, cracked nails and droopy eyes. Basically you look like poo. There is no vibrancy or beauty to you. Avoiding this is easy…sleep, sleep and more sleep.

A few years ago I had a huge muscle repair job that needed attention. I tried the Group Power class at my gym for the first time ever. It is an hourlong weightlifting class that's pretty intense. I thought I could keep up with most of the class so I loaded up my bar and off I went. I felt great at the end of the hour and I decided that I would be back in a couple of days. Well, one week later I was still sore. I had muscle aches in places where I didn't know I had muscles. I know my body worked overtime that week to repair all of the little tears I had created. Sleep is what pulled me through. Even though it took a week to repair my body, it probably would have taken two weeks if I were sleep-deprived.

Sleep is the cheapest plastic surgery you can have. Remind your partner of that when you go to bed to get your eight hours.

BENEFIT #5

FOR SLEEPING IS REDUCED HUNGER!

OK, sign me up! If hunger is directly related to too little sleep then watch out because I'm crawling in for my eight hours. This is hands down the easiest thing to do – as long as you don't talk yourself out of it.

Remember, sometimes the short goal really does benefit the long-term goal. Even if you have a million things you could do, stop and sleep. All of those 'things' will be there the next day and you can tackle them even better when you're well rested.

I went for eight years without sleeping through the night because of my daughter's diabetes. Believe me when I tell you that the next day is half as enjoyable as a day when you've had a full night's rest. Mine was unavoidable, but most people can avoid a short night's sleep by putting in a conscious effort.

When you don't sleep enough, you produce more of the appetite-stimulating hormone, ghrelin, and less of the satiety or fullness hormones, Peptide YY3-36 and leptin. So yes, there is a biological reason behind all of this. The body is an amazing machine as long as you treat it with respect and give it what it needs. As I state throughout this book, LISTEN TO YOUR BODY.

Eating salads and soups before dinner will stop the ghrelin from being released by your stomach and consequently you will feel fuller faster and eat less. If there is less ghrelin to be released, because you are sleeping enough, then this reaction will happen faster and you should eat less.

Eating slowly also will allow your brain to catch up with your stomach. There are all sorts of receptors that connect different body parts. The stomach and the brain talk to each other continually, but with a delay. It usually takes 15-20 minutes for your brain to realize there's food coming in. This is related to hormones and to blood sugar.

When my daughter has a low blood sugar she will have 15-20 grams of carbohydrates and wait 15 minutes. If her blood sugar has not risen to normal after 15 minutes, she will have 15 more grams of carbohydrates.

Lastly, research has shown that too little sleep will make you crave carbohydrates the next day. And unfortunately this usually means bad, processed, sugary, fat-laden, calorie-dense carbs. Since the body has not had sufficient time to 'reset' itself, it looks for a quick energy fix. High-calorie carbohydrates are its go-to quick energy fix food. This is not something we want to feel during the day, it really can feel like torture.

You can figure out how much sleep you require with a little experiment. Go to bed at the same time every night for two or three days and do not set an alarm clock. Wake up naturally, add up the total number of hours slept, and divide by the number of days. This will give you your sleep average. Try very hard to stick to this number, no matter what. Don't let hunger weigh you down when you can do one thing to avoid it.

Can you see how one tiny little thing like sleep can affect you in so many ways? Even though the body seems like it has individual systems, in one way or another they are all linked. This is why it is so vital to keep up your end of the deal. 'Feeding' it with these 7 A.W.E.S.O.M.E. steps will keep your wellness at its peak. Fudging on sleep really is a big deal so take it seriously.

BENEFIT #6

FOR SLEEPING IS RELAXATION!

When I have a solid night's sleep, I definitely feel relaxed, calm and cool the next day. I am able to go about my day in an organized way and not feel overwhelmed. It's hard to believe that your day can be mapped out this way just from a good night's sleep, but I know for me it's true.

When someone in our house is not being particularly friendly in the morning I say, "Wow, you woke up on the wrong side of the bed today." This morning temperament immediately sets the tone for chaos. I don't know why but then everything seems rushed and out of sorts.

Teens are notorious for not getting enough sleep during the week. Unfortunately for them, their clocks are completely opposite from the school schedule. A teen's sleep clock is more like midnight to 9 a.m., not 9 p.m. to 6 a.m.! Forget first period at 7:17 a.m.. There are a lot of school districts that have reversed the high school and elementary schedules, but so far our county has not. Thanks.

I like to begin my relaxation the night before with a pre-sleep ritual. I feel like this will carry me over to the next day and continue into my calm, cool and collected day.

Step one is I always make sure the kitchen is clean and the family room is not a total disaster before going upstairs for the night. And believe me it can become a total disaster in as little as one day. If I feel like I have the downstairs organized, then I know in the morning at 6am I will be able to function for making lunches and breakfasts for the preschool morning mayhem that occurs every day.

Do you see how this connects to sleep relaxation? It all follows the path of having things off your mind so you can sleep. A racing mind is not a mind that will fall asleep easily. Knowing that you have to do the dishes before getting the kids off to school will ultimately not make you rest very well.

Step two is organizing my day via a list for the next day. I like to look at my personal and business calendar and make a priority list. Then when the house is quiet and I can start my work, I know exactly what to do first and I don't waste any time. If you're like me, you have no time to waste.

The best organizational tool I use for my business is a weekly whiteboard. I write two to three action items the night before, sometimes with a time next to them (yes I use a timer), and then if I don't complete a task I can easily move it to the next day. My board has a notes section on the left side of the days where I can keep an ongoing list of not-so-important action items. I use mine for my business, but it would be great for personal use, too.

Step three is to get in bed to read after I've washed my face and done that routine. Reading always relaxes me and puts me to sleep, sometimes too fast because I never seem to get through my magazines or books.

Now in my head I can function the next day from morning to night. Just in case I miss writing something on my white board, I keep a pad of paper and pen in my nightstand drawer. I can quickly grab the notepad and jot down my thought so I don't have to try and remember it until morning. Relax, free up your mind and enjoy your slumber. What's your relaxation sleep ritual?

Can you believe something as easy as sleep will help you get to your healthy weight and AWESOME dream-life? Nice!

THE FIFTH SECRET TO FINDING YOUR A.W.E.S.O.M.E. IS ORGANIZATION!

Organization is extremely important when you are ready to make a change in your life, especially with food.

If you have junk food in your house you will be tempted to eat it, and if you don't have good food in your house it will be very hard to make healthy meals. It's not rocket science, it's simply that simple.

So if you are truly committed to making a change to healthy eating and living, you must organize not only your kitchen, but also the rest of your life. When you feel disorganized you will be unlikely to have the motivation to move forward on your lifestyle change. You will get overwhelmed and quit.

Organization gives you control and control is what will make you successful.

If organization doesn't come naturally to you, don't panic. It CAN be learned with a little guidance and tools. If you make up your mind to put forth the effort, I promise you it will pay off.

Here are your seven areas to organize. It really can be addicting, so if you find yourself going deeper and deeper, have fun with it and let it happen. Your life will run much smoother, I promise.

AREA #1

FOR ORGANIZATION IS YOUR PANTRY!

Step number one is to clear out the junk food in your pantry. Pack it up and give it to a homeless shelter, take it in to your or your husband's work and share it with co-workers, or hide it in another room. Whatever you choose, just get rid of it. I know it's painful, but it's such a huge help.

Then shop for good food and organize your pantry shelves by keeping like items together so you know exactly what's in there and you can do a quick scan when preparing dinner or going shopping.

This is how I organize my pantry…

Top Shelf One: baking supplies like flour, sugar, almond meal

Shelf Two: brown rice cakes and other gluten-free healthy crackers, gluten-free oats, nuts, unsweetened dried fruit, organic corn tortilla chips

Shelf Three: salsa, olives, condiments, canned fish, pasta sauce, canned tomatoes, natural nut butter, green chilis

Shelf Four: quinoa, oils (olive, sesame, grapeseed), vinegar (balsamic, rice), gluten-free pasta, vegetable broth

Floor: extra baggies and foil (all sizes), extra coffee (I buy it on sale), backup for your most used items

If this seems too basic, think again – it's supposed to be. This way you have very few temptations when you look in the pantry for something to eat. By not having cookies and other junk staring at you, it forces you to make a healthy snack or meal. It may seem boring, but it will seriously get you started down the right path.

If you must have some 'kid food' in the house, then find a different place for it besides the pantry. When my daughter makes cookies or cupcakes I tell her to hide them. She usually puts them in the dining room out of sight and I forget about them. This may seem strange, but it really works. Out of sight equals out of mind.

AREA #2

FOR ORGANIZATION IS YOUR FREEZER!

Follow the same steps for your freezer as you did with your pantry. Clear out, shop and then organize like items together for fast reference.

Here's what I keep in my freezer…(all organic, non-gmo, high quality)

- cooked chicken and shrimp
- raw chicken, shrimp, fish (salmon, mackerel, cod)
- turkey burgers, salmon burgers, ground turkey breast
- veggies (organic mix, organic edamame, broccoli, green beans)
- fruit (organic berries)
- bread and bagels (non-gmo gluten-free)

If you want more of a variety of whole foods in your freezer then go for it. I keeps things simple, which works for me. Just remember – no junk. Lean meats, veggies, whole-grain breads and fruit are the way to go.

I did keep a few frozen dinners in there for when my children needed quick meals. Trader Joe's has some decent frozen meals like fish, chicken, shepherd pie and mini tacos. These do come in handy every once in a while and I recommend having a few healthy choices in there that are microwaveable.

AREA #3

FOR ORGANIZATION IS YOUR REFRIGERATOR!

Follow the same steps for your refrigerator as you did with your pantry and freezer. Clear out, shop and then organize like items together for fast reference.

Here's what I keep in my refrigerator...

- vegetables of every color and greens (lettuce, kale)
- hummus
- unsweetened organic soy milk
- organic free range eggs
- organic sprouted tofu
- condiments (ketchup, mustard, olive oil salad dressing, organic mayo, etc...)
- fresh berries (in season)
- olives

Leftovers are a big part of your fridge, too. I always cook once and eat two or three times. Having leftovers available for your children is always a good idea. They can reheat in the microwave for a good healthy snack or meal.

Here's my Trader Joe's shopping list. This is a great tool if you want to save a lot of time. Keep a copy on your refrigerator and a highlighter close by. When you are running low on a staple, simply highlight the item and take your list with you on your shopping day. Having the list by sections makes it easy to shop aisle by aisle and not miss a thing. Happy shopping!

Shopping List - Trader Joe's

PRODUCE	sunflower seeds	TOMATOES – canned
kale	walnut pieces	*diced & fire-roasted
broccoli	peanuts	*diced no salt added
brussels sprouts	Just Mango	NUT BUTTER unsalted
spinach	New Zealand apple rings	*almond
dark lettuce	pitted prunes	*peanut
baby carrots	figs	*sunflower
long carrots	raisins	*cashew
asparagus	GROCERY	organic veg broth
green beans	black beans	just almond meal
onions	refried black beans	gluten-free oats
mushrooms	red kidney beans	REFRIGERATOR
cauliflower	Cuban-style black beans	unsweetened soy milk
bok choy	green chilis	organic eggs
sweet potatoes	salsa autentica	ground turkey breast
bell peppers	Kalamata olives	FREEZER
scallions	black olives	just chicken – cooked
tomatoes	capers	chicken tenderloins – raw
celery	organic brown rice	FISH frozen
organic tofu	organic quinoa	*salmon
beets	toasted sesame oil	*cod
lentils - steamed	grapeseed oil	turkey burgers
hummus	balsamic vinegar	salmon burgers
Medjool dates	olive oil	shrimp
apples	soy sauce gluten-free	shelled edamame
oranges	crushed garlic	organic corn
pears	Aioli garlic mustard	petite peas

kiwi	ketchup	FRUIT frozen
berries	yellow mustard	*very cherry blend
bananas	reduced fat mayonnaise	*blueberries
lemon	FISH canned	*berry medley
grapes	*yellowfin tuna	*mango
lime	*sardines	SNACKS and BREAD
avocados	*sockeye salmon	organic popping corn
fresh ginger	*smoked herring	Lundberg brown rice cakes
NUTS & DRIED FRUIT	PASTA SAUCE No Sugar	organic white corn chips
Unsweetened, Unsulfured	*Arabiata	Quinoa & black bean tortilla chips
raw almonds	*Puttanesca	soy & flaxseed tortilla chips
raw pistachios	*marinara	flaxseed meal
raw sliced almonds	garlic sea salt w/ grinder	brown rice tortillas & corn

AREA #4

FOR ORGANIZATION IS USING AN ONLINE CALENDAR!

I have no idea why I was so nervous when I made the switch to an online calendar, but it must have been that old habits die hard. There was no other logical reason, simply that I had used a paper calendar for years and it felt comforting to always have it with me.

Now I will never, ever return to paper for Google is my hero. I use gmail and Google calendar and I love having everything in one place.

The other great thing about Google calendar is that you can share your calendar with others. So if your family is running in all directions, like mine did, sharing your calendars can help keep your house somewhat under control.

Lastly, Google calendar can send you text message reminders. This has saved me many times by reminding me of an appointment. I used to think all of this was overkill, but once I got used to having the reminders, it freed up my brain tremendously. There's enough in your head so purge and feel the freedom.

Remember Secret A, Key #1, it is keeping your brain alive by putting fun stuff on your calendar. So now that you're online with your calendar, fill it up and have fun sharing it with your husband or partner. Go out there and tear up the town!

AREA #5

FOR ORGANIZATION IS STORAGE ROOMS, CLOSETS, KITCHEN CABINETS AND GARAGE!

Oh, those dreaded 'throw all' rooms. "I'll just toss it in now and organize later." How many times have you said that? And then said, "Now where did I put that?"

So here's the problem with not taking time upfront to organize storage rooms, closets and garages. It takes MORE time to find something in the mess than the time it would have taken to put it away neatly and thoughtfully. Immediate gratification of getting something out of the way will come back to haunt you when you spend an hour looking for the item later.

So you're probably asking, "What in the heck does organizing a closet have to do with getting to my healthy weight and finding my AWESOME dream-life?" Well, here's the deal. When habits are forming (as in better nutrition), it's good to form similar habits in the other areas of your life so you feel completely balanced, and you're using your time as efficiently as possible.

Here's an example. If you're starting to pack lunches and snacks so that you eat out less, you will need supplies in which to pack your food. If your kitchen is a mess and you can't find containers or a lunch box, then your packing up will become very stressful. And then if you need a cooler, which you store in the garage and the garage is a disaster, you will then have another fit looking for it.

Having everything at your fingertips is critical. Quick, efficient and low stress is the ultimate goal with everything you do, so why not start with the basics and get organized on the outside? As the outside comes together, the inside will quickly follow.

Right now I'm pretty sure you're rolling your eyes reading this thinking, "there's no way I have time to organize my whole house!" Well, you're right, you can't do it all at once, and that's why I recommend having a system to organize a little along over the next two to three months.

Step one is to prioritize your areas. If your kitchen cabinets are a mess, definitely start there.

Step two is to schedule the cleanout day on your calendar (your new Google calendar, I hope).

Step three is to put the next room on your list on your calendar in the next two to three weeks after the first cleanout day. And so forth after that.

If you spread out your cleanouts and actually put them on your calendar, you will have everything organized in no time and you won't dread it.

The key is to do a little along and look at the weather. If nasty rain is in the forecast, put a cleanout room on your calendar. You can avoid the rain blues by accomplishing a great task.

Lastly, the two best tools I like are open shelves and large clear, plastic bins. You can buy adjustable wire shelving at your local hardware store for not much money, and the clear bins are always on sale at one of the big-box stores.

The advantage of shelving and clear bins is that you have a visual on everything. You also can write on the clear bins in permanent marker and know every item that's in them.

I have four large bins for my Christmas decorations and I have them marked so I know specifically what's in them. One is lights, another is ornaments, etc...you get the idea. But because they are clear, I know there's Christmas in there. Again, quick and easy makes you function at a high level. I can have Christmas up and down in no time at all.

My mind feels relaxed and stress-free when my surroundings are organized. I hope you find the benefit to organizing your life and feeling the joy of alignment too.

AREA #6

FOR ORGANIZATION IS LISTS AND OFFICES!

Making lists is the best way to free up space in your mind. I don't know about you, but I have way too much in my head by now and I'm starting to purge. And yes, sometimes I'm purging information by accident, which is one more, very good reason to make lists.

I've already shared my shopping list with you, but I also have personal lists and work lists.

For my personal lists I keep three magnetic pads of paper on my refrigerator. List one is for the grocery, list two is for Target, list three is for random items that I get somewhere else like Sam's Club, Safeway or the pharmacy.

My children have caught on to my lists and do a fairly good job of getting items on the proper list. It's never too early to teach them organization skills.

In my business office I have a handy whiteboard on the wall with the days of the week on it and that's where I write my list for the day. There is a notes section on the left side and I can write low-priority items there. I found this board in my daughter's room (I think she bought it at 5 Below a while ago) and I quickly sucked it up since the novelty had worn off for her.

The other inexpensive tool I use for business and personal office organization is folders. I use hanging folders and plain tab folders. Hanging folders are best for storing items that you use infrequently and tab folders are great for frequent use. The tab folders now come in all colors so you can color code your desk. I use pencil to write on the tabs because then I can reuse and relabel easily.

To keep the tab folders organized, I use four standup slotted holders. Two are for business, one is personal (bills to pay and personal follow up items), and the fourth is for blank paper and sticky notes of all sizes.

Sometimes walking around an office supply store, like Office Depot, can give you really great ideas for organization. Make a list before you go of an area that needs help, and then search for ideas while you're in the store.

Organize and feel the bliss.

AREA #7

FOR ORGANIZATION IS MEALS!

OK, now we're talking nutrition. I know it sounds like a lot of preliminary work, but believe me it will pay off. Now that your entire life is more organized, you can easily take the last step, which is meal organization.

There are a couple of different parts to meal organization.

Before you organize what you're going to eat, you first have to find out what you're eating. So step one is keeping a food diary for up to one week. This can be a pain, however, it will give you a ton of information.

I recommend eating three square meals a day. The time between meals allows your body to burn your next meal efficiently. If I don't eat my three balanced meals (protein, good carb and healthy fat), then I feel unsatisfied. Feeling unsatisfied or not satiated will lead me down the wrong eating path for the entire day.

So I highly recommend keeping a food diary for at least three days (one week is better) so you can track the following in your meals:

- calories, fat, protein, carbs
- time of day
- how you feel before you eat (starving, getting hungry, your mood)
- how you feel two hours after you eat

When you evaluate your diary you probably will start to see patterns. These patterns may be good, but they also may be bad. This data will allow you to make changes. Am I eating too many carbs without protein? Do I have some healthy fat in there to help keep me satiated? Am I eating way too many calories? Am I eating when I'm stressed? Am I eating when I'm bored? Am I eating when I'm tired because I had too little sleep the night before? There are so many reasons that we eat – other than hunger. Be honest and deliberate with your diary and I promise it will pay off.

Step two is thinking about what you're going to eat ahead of time. This is important so you don't make a hasty, bad decision when you are starving. Having prepared food in the refrigerator that you can quickly grab is a lifesaver.

The weekend is a great time to prepare for the week. You don't have to spend eight hours doing this, but maybe three to four hours total over the weekend, between shopping and cooking, will be enough to give you an organized week.

Decide on the meals for the week and add any ingredients to your list that you don't have on hand. Go shopping and make sure all your staples are stocked. Cook a few things on Sunday that will last you until Wednesday. Leftovers are great for lunches and when you need to eat under a time crunch.

For me and for most parents, the nightly sports can be a killer. Practice starting at 6pm can really screw up dinner. I liked to cook on non-sport nights so that leftovers could be eaten by anyone at any time on a sport night. This was a great habit for me and it worked well. And because I eat a lot of salads for dinner and they take a while to eat, sometimes I would dump one in a large container and take it with me. I found this to be more relaxing than trying to shovel lettuce in my mouth and run out the door.

My favorite taco meat is loaded with healthy protein, beans and veggies. Adding all of the other ingredients easily turns one pound of meat into two and ups its healthiness. This would last us two to three days.

HEALTHY TACO MEAT

- 1 pound ground turkey breast

- 1 block organic sprouted tofu
- 1 bag organic frozen corn
- 2 cans petite diced tomatoes
- 1 can green chilies
- 2 cans black beans (rinsed)
- 2 tablespoons chili powder
- 1 teaspoon cumin
- 1 teaspoon paprika
- Ground red pepper to taste

Brown the ground turkey. Crumble the tofu with a fork. Add all other ingredients. Bring to a boil and then simmer for 15 minutes or until the liquid has cooked off. Enjoy!

Remember, organization is a choice. You can choose to do a little upfront work or you can run around constantly like a chicken with its head cut off.

Don't overwhelm yourself by having to organize everything all at once. Take baby steps and use this chapter as a guide. Check off the areas you get done and you will feel relief each time you start the next step. You can do it!

THE SIXTH SECRET TO FINDING YOUR A.W.E.S.O.M.E. IS BEING MINDFUL!

STEP #1

FOR BEING MINDFUL IS FORGETTING THE SMALL STUFF!

Forgetting the small stuff is easier said than done for me. I tend to be a perfectionist so I'm all about the small stuff. I literally work on this daily, because it does not come naturally to me. The good news, if you follow me in this perfectionist world, is that with hard work you can modify your ways and change for the better.

When I became a single parent is when I really started to notice that I didn't, one, have time for the small stuff, and two, think the small stuff was important anymore.

The more I ran around like a chicken with my head cut off, the more I realized that if I didn't slow down and enjoy my children (and my life), I would miss out on everything and then I would be too old to enjoy anything. Thus, the only way to slow down is to let some things go; i.e. the small stuff.

So what is the small stuff? I guess it's slightly different for everyone, but here are some things I do a lot less frequently: polishing the silver candlesticks for the holidays (seriously who does that?), putting up outside holiday decorations, not cooking the entire holiday meal myself, vacuuming the entire house perfectly every week (now I have a cordless vacuum for quick dog hair pickup), putting my children's clean clothes away for them (now they get dressed out of a laundry basket), keeping the basement perfect (it's their space so they live with the mess), etc....You get the idea.

These details did not interfere with the organization of my house, they simply took time. This was all time that I wanted to spend elsewhere. If your small stuff can disappear without anyone noticing, then it probably didn't need to be there in the first place.

What are some details that you can let go? If you put some thought to it, I bet you will come up with a list of five or six. Give it a try and see how liberating it feels.

STEP #2

FOR BEING MINDFUL IS IGNORING GOSSIP AND DRAMA!

This one can be very challenging for many people, especially now with all of the social media out there.

What I tell my children is "gossip and drama breeds gossip and drama". It's extremely simple. If you want to lead a drama-free life then stay out of the drama.

The words gossip and drama mean negativity and hurtfulness to me. So the next question is, why do people want to be negative and hurtful? There are only two words to answer that and they are lack of self-confidence and jealousy.

The next questions are what is lack of self-confidence and why are people jealous? Well, the simple answer is they're not tough enough to go out and get what they want in life because they are afraid of failure.

Very successful people make a ton of mistakes along the way to their success. Then how are they successful, you ask? They are successful because they learn from their mistakes, make changes and most importantly, never give up. If you get discouraged from your mistakes and give up, then you'll never achieve the success you desire.

Here's a simple example. My daughter trained a very young, off the track thoroughbred horse for free. This is called a free lease because you pay only for the board and you can return the horse at any time.

When she got Luna (the horse) all she could do was walk, trot and canter. She would stop dead at the gate of the ring when Julia was on her because she missed her field mates and she wanted to stop working. Julia had the hardest time trying to make her walk past the gate. She persisted, and after a few weeks of doing what her trainer told her to do, Luna finally stopped that bad behavior. After a few months Julia trained her to jump a 2' course in the ring, and when she took her to her very first horse show Luna completed the entire course.

So you're probably saying, "Wow, good for her," just like most mature people would say. Well, the problem was that people at her barn were not saying that. They said things like "Julia's not a good enough rider to train that horse" and "Look, she can't even get her to go past the gate, geez what's wrong with her?"

Julia would get in the car in tears because of all the gossip going on that she could hear plain as day. The girls didn't even try to be quiet about it. So as I told her, "Not one of those girls at that barn would dare set foot on that baby race horse, they are all jealous of you. They don't have the guts you have or the self-confidence to do what you're doing."

Now this was a very hard concept for a 13-year-old because all she cared about was fitting in and being liked, but when Luna really started to excel at her training I think Julia started to see it from my point of view. And by the way, Luna took care of Julia for months and never dumped her. She didn't buck or take off. They were an amazing pair.

So as you can see, lack of self-confidence and jealousy are behind most gossip and drama. If those girls had self-confidence in their riding abilities, then they would not have been picking on my daughter. Find your comfortable place and don't worry about others. You will be much happier.

STEP #3

FOR BEING MINDFUL IS PICKING A MANTRA (OR TWO)!

What the heck is a mantra and why do I need one?

A mantra is defined in the dictionary as "an often repeated word, formula, or phrase, often a truism." I like to use mantras to get me through a difficult or stressful time.

A few of my favorites are:

- "This too shall pass"
- "Keep going"
- "I can do it"
- "Relax"

When I'm facing a challenging situation, I'm nervous, or I'm in a difficult cycle of my life, I like to 'chant' one of these phrases to myself continually. Mind over matter and having a positive outlook will usually make for a positive result. I truly believe this and it works.

In the span of two years my daughter was diagnosed with Type I diabetes, both of my children were diagnosed with celiac, I got divorced, and my ex-husband moved to California. Believe me, I used all four of my mantras all day every day for a while there. They really worked. I simply got up each day and continued on. Dwelling can cause you to crumble and fail. Tell yourself you can do something, this too shall pass, and keep going.

I definitely believe everyone needs a mantra or two because they help keep you focused and positive. Life changes on a daily basis so if you persevere and put one foot in front of the other you will eventually get where you want to go. Your mind is the most powerful organ in your body. Tell yourself you are capable of success and you will be successful. It's really that easy.

STEP #4

FOR BEING MINDFUL IS CHANGING COURSE WHEN HEADING FOR THE REFRIGERATOR!

So you've had 'one of those days' where everything goes wrong and everyone awoke on the wrong side of the bed. Or maybe it's just kind of 'blah, normal' and you're bored. Some days just aren't great and you have to deal with them.

But how do you deal with a bad day? Do you go home and raid the pantry or refrigerator? The answer for most of us is yes! Emotional eating is very common and that crazy dopamine hormone that's released is why. The more fat, sugar and salt you have the better you feel. Well, temporarily that is. Food is immediate gratification and the only thing we want immediately after a bad day is to feel better.

My answer to this is to replace the immediate gratification of food, with another activity that you really enjoy. Sometimes when we replace something, we don't miss it as much.

Think of an activity that you enjoy that could take the place of food. Some suggestions are taking the dog for a walk, biking around your neighborhood, calling your best friend, watching a favorite show that you have recorded, writing in a journal, playing with your children, knitting, reading or taking a relaxing bath with an aromatic candle.

When you choose an activity, post it in your kitchen on the pantry and refrigerator doors. Mine is 'food or bike ride?' This may sound strange, but it does work. The note reminds you to be mindful of your eating. Are you really hungry or are you emotionally (bored, sad, mad) eating?

When you start to ask yourself this question every time you reach for food, your mind and body will finally be in alignment. This alignment is one key toward reaching your ultimate goal of health, happiness, and your healthy weight.

STEP #5

FOR BEING MINDFUL IS BEING THANKFUL!

I know I can forget to be thankful, can you?

It's so easy to go about your day and forget what you DO have. We all are programmed to want more, but not programmed to be thankful for what we have. Why is this? How did our world become so materialistic? Shall I list all of the holidays filled with 'things' – Halloween, Christmas, Easter, Hanukkah and birthdays are what come to my mind, but I'm sure there are more.

I'm not saying 'things' are bad, I'm simply saying that we can't forget to be thankful for what really matters in life – your health, your family's health and the love and laughter you share with friends and family.

My life did not turn out as I had planned in my head – diabetes, celiac, divorce and ex-husband relocation - were not part of it; but regardless of those difficulties, the way I look at life now, as opposed to then, has been the most dramatic and best change ever.

I'm pretty sure I had an ongoing competition with myself when I graduated from college. It went something like this, now I have to...get a job and make a decent living, get married, have children (a boy and a girl), drive a cool car, get a dog, live in a nice house, party every weekend with other cool parents, and who knows what else... and then I'll be happy. Or so I thought!

Now I look at my life years later and laugh. How wrong and idealistic could I have been? That materialistic world I was living in was not the real me. The real me is a mom who secretly liked being a taxi driver and who loves watching her children thrive. I loved living at either the hockey rink or the horse barn. I drove my same car for 15 years and cried when it died.

So now I'm just thankful and grateful. Love, laughter and vacation. That's all I need.

STEP #6

FOR BEING MINDFUL IS SEEKING HELP FOR DEPRESSION!

I wish depression weren't such a taboo subject. It's real and it's common and if you have signs of depression you need to ask for help. An evaluation by a qualified doctor can help determine if you have situational depression (brought on by something like divorce), clinical depression (the inherited kind) or if you are having a sensitivity to something else like a food or a medication.

It's not one-stop shopping when it comes to depression, but the good news is that whatever kind of depression you have, there is help out there. Medication can help short-term with situational depression or long-term with clinical depression. If you think you are having a drug interaction, make sure you share that information with the specialist. Lastly, food sensitivities can cause depression like symptoms. Gluten, dairy and sugar are the most common, but there are many more possibilities. An elimination diet can help you figure out to what foods you may be sensitive.

Somewhere in time, mental illness has received a bad rap. The brain is the most complicated, amazing organ in our body and we don't give it enough attention. Things can go wrong in the brain and it's of no fault to the person. Depression is no different than any other disease.

If my daughter doesn't take her insulin every day, she will die. If someone with a mental illness doesn't take medication she can die. There's no difference in my book. Accept and treat the illness you have and move on with your life.

I know when I was going through my bad years I had situational depression. I slept all the time, I felt like I was frowning constantly, I didn't want to socialize and I just didn't feel like my normal happy self. I tried a medication for a few months, but for me I just had to get through my bad cycle. I think the medication took the 'edge off', but as time went on I started to feel better naturally.

If you feel like you struggle through each day I strongly urge you to take that first step, which can be the hardest, and make an appointment with a doctor who can evaluate you. You have one life to live and I say rock it the best you can. Whether you need medication or not, feeling the best you can feel every day is the ultimate goal. If you need medication, then you do. If it's situational, then time will heal you. If it's food or another drug, then a food elimination or a drug change can take care of it. There are many possibilities so reach out to someone and feel your best.

STEP #7

FOR BEING MINDFUL IS LAUGHTER!

Laughter really is the best medicine. How many times have you heard that?

Serotonin, your natural antidepressant hormone, is released when you laugh so you're getting your medicine without even knowing it. No pills or potions, just naturally occurring hormones. Now that's cool.

Over the years I've definitely changed my tv watching to funny sitcoms. I used to watch a bunch of dramas, but I found myself not enjoying them anymore. Now when I sit down for a show I want to laugh and relax.

Sometimes just smiling can do the trick. Try this experiment. Smile and hold it for 15 seconds. Do you feel the tension release on your face? Are you smiling even bigger now because you feel silly for smiling?

Our lives can get so involved on most days that we forget to enjoy the tiny things around us. Take a minute to find something that can make you smile and do this a couple of times a day. My dog makes me smile every day. I have a pitbull mix named Bauer. We got him from the SPCA and he's been a great dog. He has an underbite and every time I look at him I smile.

What in your life makes you smile every day? Maybe it's a pet, a funny tv show, a funny YouTube video or your children. Whatever it is, find it, smile, laugh and feel great.

STEP #8

FOR BEING MINDFUL IS BEING POSITIVE!

I know I've talked a lot about this already, but I cannot stress enough the importance of thinking positively. A positive attitude will result in a positive outcome. It works. I promise.

The mind is unbelievably powerful and when it's connected to your body and you're aligned, you will be successful.

I'm not saying you won't have any bumps or bruises along the way, I'm simply saying that if you stay the course and believe that the ultimate outcome will be positive, then it will be. I know for me I've had to test this theory many times, and I still test it daily. I use my positive mantras all the time to keep me focused.

Doubt, aka the little devil on our shoulder, can be the problem. When we're thinking positively and we're doing all the right things and life still isn't going in the right direction, it's very easy to doubt yourself and get down. I know these last years for me as a business owner have been a huge rollercoaster. I'm up, I'm down, I'm up, I'm down...I'm going to succeed, I'm not going to succeed...this business stinks, this business rocks... my children are awesome, my children are from hell...blah, blah, blah.

So bye, bye little devil on my shoulder, as I knock you off one last time. I will succeed, my business does rock and my children are (mostly) awesome. You will not make me doubt myself because I am stronger than you.

Mind over matter does work. However, it can be hard, it can be annoying, and it can be daily. Like anything, however, positive thinking can become habitual. The more you do it, the more natural it becomes.

Here's a fun example of how I used a positive thinking mantra to get me through a sticky situation. One summer Stephen and I went whitewater rafting. Instead of going in the four-man raft with a guide, we used the single-person blow up kayaks called duckies. Even though I had only been whitewater rafting one time when I was 13 in the big raft, I agreed to try the ducky. Off we go in the rapids. We're both doing really well until we get to the class 4 'single-person slot', as the guide called it. He told us most people fall out at this rapid; and proceeded to tell us to go feet first in the water if we do fall out because it's safer, and then swim to the side, and hopefully recover our ducky not too far downstream.

I was in front of Stephen and as I started to see the 'slot' my heart started to race, I clenched my teeth and I immediately started to repeat to myself, "I can do it." I must have repeated it at least 50 times even though 'the slot' was all of a 10-second ride. I made it and just as I turned around to watch Stephen, out he went! Now we do tend to be slightly competitive with each other so believe me I have enjoyed that one for a very long time. Who knows why I made it through that rapid? Some say beginners' luck, but I will always believe it was my positive thinking. I told myself I was going to do something and I did it. Use it, live it, love it and enjoy the success.

STEP #9

FOR BEING MINDFUL IS NOT TO WORRY!

What exactly is worry? The definition from Wikipedia is "thoughts, images and emotions of a negative nature in which mental attempts are made to avoid anticipated potential threats." If you read it like I do, "mental attempts" is the key here. Mentally you want to change something, but it's not possible to mentally make a physical change in someone or something else if you're not physically present.

So what exactly does worry accomplish? If it's thoughts and emotions, but no action, then how are you going to change the outcome? The answer is, you're not. I can worry all day about how my daughter's diabetes is doing while she's in school, but since I am not with her and I have no way of asking her, then why worry? How does it make the situation better? There's no way I can change an outcome with her diabetes simply by giving it negative mental energy.

Now I'm not saying you don't plan and take precautionary steps prior to an event. Of course she has glucose tablets and her blood meter with her at all times. She even has backup supplies in the nurse's office at school. So given that she has her supplies and knows what to do, my worry is fruitless. Do you see the difference? Once a plan has been made and the event is occurring, you have to let it go and hope for the best. That's where that positive thinking comes in – again. Geez, see how it creeps in everywhere?

Worry also can set you up for anxiety issues. Anxiety wreaks havoc on the body in many physical ways. You can have irritability, restlessness, insomnia, heart palpitations, headaches, muscle tension, shortness of breath, sweaty palms, nausea, and dizziness, just to name a few. If you don't want to reach the point of anxiety, then STOP the worry! You can 'train' yourself not to worry by using your mantras. Pick a mantra, such as "stop worrying, it does no good, relax," and repeat it to yourself as much as necessary. Slowly the worry will be less and less.

Organizing and planning will help keep worry to a minimum. Try not to live 'by the seat of your pants'. This will only set you up for worry because you will concentrate on everything you could have done to prevent a disaster. Once you feel you've done everything possible for a situation, move on and put your energy into your next project. Your body will respond by feeling relaxed and aligned.

In my opinion, this is the hardest secret. Daily physical tasks can leave me feeling 'brain dead' by the end of the day and I 'forget' to be mindful. Make a conscious effort to reverse this and take time for yourself (like early morning yoga) before starting your crazy, busy day. You will notice a huge difference in how you feel throughout the day.

THE SEVENTH SECRET TO FINDING YOUR A.W.E.S.O.M.E. IS ENVISIONING AND LIVING YOUR TRUE LIFE!

So right now you're possibly saying, "It doesn't matter what my true life is, this is the life I have been given." Well, I'm here to tell you...that's not true! You can design your life if you believe you can design your life.

If you can envision it, you can live it.

Here are some steps to help you start living your true life the way you want to live it. Start by answering the following steps truthfully. The truth is always the beginning of success.

STEP #1

FOR ENVISIONING AND LIVING YOUR TRUE LIFE IS LOOKING AT YOUR PHYSICAL SELF!

So I know you're reading this book to reach your healthy weight, gain energy, and start living your AWESOME dream-life, but have you looked at the rest of you recently? I don't mean to sound petty, but our physical self plays a large part in our confidence level. When we look good, we feel good. It's plain and simple and every female out there knows this.

Have you had a new 'hair-do' lately? Maybe your hair style has been the same for 20 years and you really could use a new style. Just do it, it's only hair. If you hate the new cut, then you always can go back to the old style. Is the gray starting to bother you, but you're not into dyeing your hair? Ask your hairdresser for some highlights or go to the drugstore and buy some highlights (that can be slightly scary, though). Sometimes highlights can hide the gray without completely changing the color. Don't be scared to update and feel 'fresh'.

Have you looked in your closet lately? Are you wearing clothes from college (and I don't mean nostalgic sweat clothes)? Do you hate to shop like I do, but you really need a few new things?

I find shopping with a friend at smaller stores like Marshalls and TJ Maxx is easier on me mentally than going to the mall. I get overwhelmed in huge department stores and end up leaving without trying on anything. I also like a bargain, so finding designer clothes for less money is always up my alley. My daughter and I like the consignment stores too. They're great for designer purses and jeans. Just a couple of new (to you) things make all the difference in the world. Classic pants and jeans last a long time so as long as you're staying current with your tops and shoes, you are good to go.

The last little tidbit is your nails. I know it may seem silly, but I feel good when my toes are done and looking hot in some fun sandals. I don't fool with painting my fingernails (I'm more of a short nail person), but I do like to keep a nice pedicure. My daughter and I will have a pedicure night. We'll soak, clip, file and paint each other's nails. Julia got me started on adding a glitter top coat or decals. One (entire) summer I had bright pink toes with pretty flower decals. I was obsessed with those flowers.

So if you've been thinking, I want my hair to look like this, I love these designer jeans, I really need some fresh clothes, and I want zippy toes in some fresh cute sandals, then just do it. Put it on your calendar and make it happen. If you can envision it, you can live it.

STEP #2

FOR ENVISIONING AND LIVING YOUR TRUE LIFE IS BEING HAPPY WITH YOUR PHYSICAL SURROUNDINGS!

Your physical surroundings are very important. I lived in my house for 20 years and I had it just the way I wanted it. It was a pit when we bought it and I worked hard to get it looking pretty. I loved coming home to such a comfortable and safe space.

However, my next house will be on the water. I know that. It's my vision and I will live it. The peacefulness of the water is extremely soothing and important to me.

What and where is your perfect house? Maybe you're in it. Maybe you're not. Take some time to think and search. I like to search online every couple of months just to see what's out there and to feel inspired.

Maybe you see yourself living in a completely different state. Do you need more heat or more cold weather? Do you like the water or mountains? Are you a city person or country?

If you've never asked these questions, then it's time you do. You may surprise yourself with the answers.

If you want to move one day, but it's not possible right now, then think about your current living situation. If you live in a single-family house then you have options not only on the inside, but on the outside as well. Come up with a plan to update. What colors are inspiring you lately? Have you always wanted a bright yellow bedroom, but you were nervous to give it a try? Just do it. It's only paint and you always can paint over it. I love paint. It is the number one way to brighten and refresh a house. And it's fairly cheap if you do it yourself.

When I was married, my husband did all of the gardening. When he moved out I was forced to take over. At first I felt overwhelmed because I had never done much outside, but then as I got started I decided I liked it. It was a great outlet on a beautiful day and when my project was complete I loved admiring my work.

Over the years I have made my gardens very easy and self-sustaining. I love perennials because they hop up year after year on their own. Hostas, ornamental grasses and flowers like iris and lilies can make your garden pop. The only maintenance is cutting them back when they die in the fall and then they're ready to go in the spring with new growth.

Comfort, peace, and serenity all can be found in your living space. Decide what resonates with you and make it your goal to create it.

STEP #3

FOR ENVISIONING AND LIVING YOUR TRUE LIFE IS CLOSELY EXAMINING YOUR RELATIONSHIP WITH YOUR SPOUSE OR PARTNER!

This could be the hardest and most important step you take. How do I look at my long-term relationship and go through it with a fine-tooth comb? Am I happy? Truly happy? Let's hope the answer is yes. But if it's not, then be honest and try to figure out why.

I want you to approach this in a positive way. First, focus on what's good with your spouse or partner and in your relationship.

Make a list and look at it. And I mean really look at it. Think, reflect and ask "Is this why I fell in love with this person?" This is very important because many times we 'forget' the good and only focus on the bad.

Second, make a list of the 'things' that you don't like in your relationship. Write them all down, big and small.

Third, scratch off incidentals. Things that 'simply don't matter'. We all have them, so be mature and ignore some tiny issues. Instead, laugh about them and make them a part of your person.

One 'thing' that bugs me about Stephen is that he has long, and I mean long, pauses when he's talking. When we first started dating I used to ask him at least 10 times per phone conversation, "are you still there?". He formulates (in paragraph style) what he's going to say in his head before spitting it out. I'm used to it now and so I just laugh about it. It's who he is and in the long run the conversations are very effective and meaningful. So I scratched that one off my list, and now I just wait patiently.

Fourth, go to your spouse with the remaining list and discuss it. You may be surprised by how many things are on your list that your partner didn't know bugged you. And have him or her do the same for you. A partnership works both ways afterall.

Lastly, if you think you need outside help, like a marriage counselor, then don't be afraid to get it. I know plenty of couples who have successfully gone to marriage counseling. A third party is always a great way to gain perspective. If counseling doesn't work and you decide to end your relationship, then you can do so knowing you gave it your best shot, and you can walk away feeling comfortable with your decision.

There are all sorts of reasons that relationships don't work. It is not black or white. I know three women who were married to men, and ended their marriages in order to live with women. Every relationship is unique. Examine yours and figure out if you are living it authentically.

STEP #4

FOR ENVISIONING AND LIVING YOUR TRUE LIFE IS EXAMINING YOUR CAREER!

Do you like your job? Do you love your job? Do you tolerate your job? Do you hate your job? Do you want a job?

So where do you fit? I used to like my job and now I love my job. It makes a big difference. I know there are a ton of good reasons that people stay in jobs; money, benefits and security come to mind. All very important and top of the list. Feeling comfortable in a familiar routine is another one. Comfortable. Hmmm...why is it so hard to step out of that comfort zone?

But what if you could live your dream job? What would it be? Have you ever thought about it?

When I ask my clients this question I usually get a long stare. And then I get a well thought out answer followed by why it would never work. Well, I'm this and there's that, and it's...scary! Yes, scary is usually the number one reason that someone doesn't pursue a passion.

Stepping out of your comfort zone can be really hard, but once you do it once it gets easier every time thereafter. Believe me, I'm out of my comfort zone on a daily basis in my business. It's definitely easier now than it used to be, but I still push myself daily. Yes, daily. Some days I'm slightly uncomfortable, but other days, say when I have to talk in front of a large group of people, I'm very uncomfortable. It's kind of like exercising. It can be hard to get started, but you always feel good when it's over. And I love my work so it's worth it.

Maybe you don't need to open your own business, like I did, but that doesn't mean you can't look around. Sign up for job board emails that pertain to your passionate field and stay in the loop as to what's out there. Send your resume around and go on interviews if you get them. Getting started is usually the hardest part to anything. This is a great way to pursue your passion without giving up your paycheck.

Lastly, if your passion is to own your own business, call me and I'll help you get started. There are so many resources out there for small business owners that you do not have to do it all on your own. The counties and states offer a ton of help. If you have the passion, energy and time, then owning your own business is extremely rewarding.

Try not to stay in a job that drains you. If you do, your wellness goals will be extremely hard to achieve and your life will not be as joyous. Spending 40 hours a week at your job is a huge hunk of your life. Try and make those hours as pleasant as possible and you will notice a huge difference in your attitude toward everything and everyone in your life.

STEP #5

FOR ENVISIONING AND LIVING YOUR TRUE LIFE IS TRAVELING!

Do you love to travel but life has you weighed down so you have put it on the back burner? Do you miss it and feel like your life is not complete?

Well, I'll answer that – yes! I've had to put my expensive travel plans on hold for some years, but that doesn't mean I stay home all the time.

Even if you can't get to the Caribbean or Europe, you can still take small trips. These small trips can be fun even if they aren't extravagant.

I highly recommend a weekend away with just your partner. A few days can rejuvenate a relationship in many ways. We've had all sorts of little weekend getaways such as Chesapeake, Maryland (the city at the very top of the Chesapeake Bay) in a B & B for a night, a Shenandoah mountain cabin (for my 40th birthday – which I don't really recommend), Atlantic City (yucky casino smoke, but kind of fun if you win), New York City (always my favorite for shows and food), Charleston, South Carolina (that was a longer trip and a lovely city), Bethany Beach and West Virginia. There are a ton of places to go within an hour or two of your house that are very affordable.

Believe it or not, I have actually talked to people who have never left their children and had a trip away by themselves. That's very unusual, and in my opinion, not very healthy. I think your relationship with your partner has to be nourished in order for it to thrive. And it's very hard to do that at your house with your children always around. I guess some can do it, but I strongly recommend planning some weekends away and enjoying your partner in peace.

One of the very best trips Stephen and I had was a free trip to France and Monaco. It was a trip through our family business, when I worked there, that was given to us when we purchased a certain amount of merchandise. Stephen and I had been dating only one year when I asked him to go, and my parents went too because it was a trip for four. It was first class all the way with five-star hotels and food. We still talk about that trip and probably will for life. And yes, traveling is very easy when you're not paying. We will always remember that time together and how important it was for us to get away from our five children. It was truly special, and something that we will always cherish.

So for me, traveling is part of who I am. I love learning about new cultures and seeing a different way of living. I appreciate and respect others and how they were raised.

The best experience of my life, culturally speaking, was when I lived in London, England, my junior year of college. I had the opportunity to live with a family and go to the University of London for my second semester. Not only did I experience the British way of living, but I was able to travel extensively. We took weekend trips all over the UK and longer trips to France, Spain, Italy, Greece, Austria and Switzerland, just to name a few. I came home with a more liberal way of thinking about other cultures and ethnicities. Traveling as a student is the cheapest way to go too. Youth hostels were a mainstay for us, and when you're young you don't really care where you sleep or what you eat.

If traveling is on your bucket list, then start small if you can't do a big trip, but I encourage you to not put it off until the children are grown. Take some small trips alone and some longer trips with your family through our county. I have seen more of Europe than my own country, which is strange. The Grand Canyon and the Northwest coast are on the top of my list. I'd like to visit every state before I die.

Travel is part of living your true life. Now get out there and plan a trip.

STEP # 6

FOR ENVISIONING AND LIVING YOUR TRUE LIFE IS EXAMINING YOUR RELIGIOUS BELIEFS OR SPIRITUALITY!

How do you feel about religion, spirituality and God? Are you comfortable with your beliefs and with your commitment? Do you feel guilty for not attending church on a regular basis? Do you want to get more involved, but you just haven't for one reason or another? Do you have different beliefs than your partner?

For many people and couples, these can be difficult questions. I grew up not attending church, but I married a religious man and my current partner, Stephen, is religious. It was a small sticky point with both of them, but over the years we have grown to respect each other's beliefs.

I would say that I am spiritual. I don't attend church on a regular basis, but I enjoy going occasionally with Stephen. I find the messages and the energy in the church very uplifting and positive. In general I think churches are wonderful. They bring people together in a positive way, they give back to the community, they provide positive weekly messages by which to live, they educate, and they offer a great social life.

The point to examining your spirituality is to make sure that you are comfortable with your beliefs. Your beliefs are what matter here, because this is all about you after all. If you feel like something is not right and you'd like to make a change, then make a list and start working on it.

Maybe the church choir needs more participants and you've always wanted to sing? Maybe they do a food drive every year and you've always thought about helping? Maybe you dislike going and you need to discuss a plan with your spouse?

Respecting others views' is always important, and it can be critical when it comes to spirituality and religion. Wars are still being fought over religion, and I'm guessing that will always be the case. Figure out what you need and go get it.

Envisioning and living your true life is the ultimate in alignment. If you've reached this level then you should feel very comfortable with who you are and with what you've accomplished in your life. Celebrate!

Congratulations! We're talking about the seven secrets to feeling A.W.E.S.O.M.E. and we have now finished every secret. Let's take a quick look at everything you've just learned.

SECRET A = ACTIVE MIND AND BODY

Key #1 is keeping your brain alive. Spice up your life by putting some fun stuff on your calendar. Do this for you, you + partner and family.

Key #2 is keeping your relationships healthy. My five relationship pieces are my partner, my parents, my sibling, my friends and my parents. If there's a conflict, work it out.

Key #3 is enjoying your children. Along with parenting, have fun with them! Laugh, ride bikes, play games – whatever is your pleasure.

Key #4 is getting involved in your community. You can get involved in your neighborhood, your city or your children's school. It makes you feel good to give back for free.

Key #5 is joining a club. There are so many out there, just pick your favorite. Knit, run, read...

Key #6 is cooking. Oh the joy of cooking. Cook some bulk items on Sunday and think simple. No recipes needed.

Key #7 is saying NO. That's right, just say no. If you are overbooked and cranky then turn something down. It's OK and it will keep you sane.

SECRET W = WHOLESOME FOODS

Food #1 is vegetables. Eat a rainbow of vegetables and a lot of them. They are high in antioxidants, high in fiber and low in calories.

Food #2 is fruit. Eat 1-2 servings a day. Fruit is high in antioxidants, high in fiber and a good carbohydrate. If you are looking for something sweet, fruit is your go-to food.

Food #3 is grains. Whole grains like quinoa are important for their protein and fiber. They will keep you satiated and give you a nice slow-burning carb for all day energy.

Food #4 is protein. Protein is important for your body to function properly all day. You need about ½ your body weight per day and protein ups your metabolism.

Food #5 is sugar. Sugar in fruit is healthy and good. Added sugar like in soda and processed foods will add calories but no nutrients. It is also very addictive!

Food #6 is fat. Most of your fat should come from plants. Second to plant fat is lean poultry, fish and eggs. Fat helps with satiety, but watch your portions because it is calorie-dense.

Food #7 is water. Water is important because it keeps you hydrated and allows your body to perform optimally. Switching to water from diet drinks can also help you get rid of a sugar addiction. Drink up before eating, because thirst mimics hunger.

Food #8 is condiments and spices. Condiments and spices are a great way to improve your health because they are loaded with antioxidants. You also can turn a boring meal into a lively meal just with a few additions from your spice rack or fridge.

SECRET E = EXERCISE

Benefit #1 is heart health. Aerobic exercise helps keep your heart muscle strong and helps lower your blood pressure. 150 minutes per week is recommended.

Benefit #2 is bone health. Weight-bearing exercises, like lifting weights, helps keep your bones strong and your balance on track. Eat calcium-rich foods like kale and sardines to help ward off osteoporosis.

Benefit #3 is calorie health. The more you exercise, the more calories you burn. The more calories you burn, the more food you can eat.

Benefit #4 is sugar health. Exercise lowers your blood sugar, which means you need less insulin. Using less insulin helps preserve your pancreas and may help delay blood sugar diseases like Type 2 diabetes.

Benefit #5 is friend, partner or me time. Motivation and laughter from a friend or partner during exercise will help keep you going on a regular basis. If you need alone time, then exercise by yourself.

Benefit #6 is brain health. Serotonin is the key to a happy brain. Exercise makes us happy, which makes us smile, which releases serotonin. This natural antidepressant keeps our brain healthy.

Benefit #7 is example setting. Your children will exercise and eat right if they see you doing it.

SECRET S = SLEEP

Benefit #1 is creating a supercharged immune system. Sleep is a great way to allow your body to reset itself and fight off any foreign invaders that are trying to make you sick. If you feel like you're getting sick, go to bed for a good 10 hours and see if you can prevent the bug from attacking you.

Benefit #2 is growing. Yes, I threw in one for our children because it's so important and I didn't want to overlook it. Growth hormones are released in the early morning, usually two hours before we wake. If your children are shorting their sleep, their growth hormones are going to be shorted as well.

Benefit #3 is brain health. The brain recharges at night and prepares for its long day the next day with plenty of sleep. The neurons connect and give us clear thinking, a good memory, happy feelings, and quick thinking.

Benefit #4 is beauty sleep. Who doesn't want this? Bright eyes, clear skin and shiny hair are just a few beauty enhancements. It's the cheapest plastic surgery out there.

Benefit #5 is reduced hunger. Sleeping enough will keep your hormones balanced and not make you crave terrible processed high-fat carbs the next day.

Benefit #6 is relaxation. Being organized before you go to sleep by having a pre-sleep ritual will allow you to have a great night's sleep, and make you feel cool, calm and collected the next day.

SECRET O = ORGANIZATION

Area #1 is your pantry. Arrange like items together and keep staples always on hand.

Area #2 is your freezer. Arrange like items together and keep staples always on hand.

Area #3 is your refrigerator. Arrange like items together and keep staples always on hand.

Area #4 is your calendar. Use an online calendar such as Google and share it with your husband or partner. Set it up so it sends you text messages and keeps you informed at all times. This will free up your brain for more fun stuff.

Area #5 is storage rooms, closets, kitchen cabinets and garage. Put one of these rooms on your calendar once a month. Pick a rainy day and get cleaning.

Area #6 is lists. Always keep staples on hand by writing them down on a list. Keep a few magnetic pads on your refrigerator so they are handy.

Area #7 is meals. Always having something healthy in the refrigerator will help keep you from eating the wrong food.

SECRET M = MINDFUL

Step #1 is forgetting the small stuff. Leave the details behind and forget being a perfectionist. The big picture with friends, family, health and happiness is what really matters.

Step #2 is ignoring gossip and drama. The best way to stay authentic to yourself is to ignore gossip and drama because it will suck you in and take you down the wrong path. If you're not gossiping, then that means you have self-confidence in who you are and what kind of life you are leading.

Step #3 is picking a mantra and using it daily. A mantra can be as simple as "I can do this" or "this too shall pass." Mind over matter plays a big role in success. Tell yourself what you want to come true, and it will.

Step #4 is changing course when heading for the refrigerator. Mindless and emotional eating are extremely common and can kill your goals. Make sure you are hungry before reaching for something to eat. If you're not, change course and go for an activity instead.

Step #5 is being thankful every day. Be thankful and grateful for what you do have and not for what you do not have. If you think the glass is half full, it will be.

Step #6 is seeking help for depression when needed. Do not be shy about asking for help if you think you are suffering with depression. Mental illness is just as real as any other disease. There are plenty of resources out there that can help you live a very normal and happy life.

Step #7 is laughing often. Laughter releases serotonin, the natural antidepressant hormone, so seek out something funny every day and get that belly laugh going. Sitcoms are a great resource.

Step #8 is thinking positively. Positive thinking creates positive results. The mind-body connection is amazing and when aligned you will notice a huge difference in your life.

Step #9 is stop worrying. The only thing worrying does is breed anxiety. Get yourself organized, come up with a plan and stop the worry. Once something is out of your control, you have to let it go.

SECRET E = ENVISIONING AND LIVING YOUR TRUE LIFE

Step #1 is looking at your physical self. Are you happy with your weight, your hair, your clothes and your nails? Feeling pretty and sassy is important so don't overlook it.

Step #2 is examining your physical surroundings. Are you happy with your house and where you live? If you need a little pick-me-up on the inside, paint is always a nice way to freshen up.

Step #3 is taking a look at your relationship with your partner. If it's not great, then take some time to talk with your partner and try to figure out how to improve it. Communication can usually fix things.

Step #4 is making sure you are happy in your career. If you're not then start to look around at different jobs. Sometimes a small change can make the difference between liking your job and loving your job. You don't always have to have a total career change to make a difference.

Step #5 is getting travel back on your list if you miss it. Sometimes the big expensive trips can't happen right away, but some smaller weekend trips can refresh you and help your relationship at the same time.

Step #6 is examining your religious beliefs and spirituality. If you've gotten out of the habit of going to church for one reason or another, and you really miss it, then put it on your calendar for the month. If you can only attend one Sunday a month, that's OK. Going every once in a while is going to make you feel better than never going. If church isn't for you, then admit it and be comfortable with your decision.

SUMMARY

Amazing! You now have the recipe for living *Your A.W.E.S.O.M.E. Life: How to Reach Your Healthy Weight and Live Your Life Feeling Energized and Balanced.* I hope you've enjoyed the journey.

Speaking of journey. Remember that "wellness is a journey and not a destination". You're never really 'done' healing, but you can get to a very comfortable place with the 7 Secrets.

So much of success is determined in your head. Telling yourself you can do something will usually result in a positive outcome. And conversely, thinking negatively will produce negative results.

Lastly, you will need to live by and practice the 7 Simple Secrets for most of your life in order to stay at the top of your dream-life. Remember...journey, not destination.

Your life is a roller coaster. Sometimes you're up and sometimes you're down. It's a series of peaks and valleys. This book is designed to help you find your peak. We all need help getting back on track sometimes, and simple steps like these can help you do that.

Remember, finding your healthy weight, gaining energy, and feeling emotionally balanced equal your dream-life. Baby steps will get you there, and if you need more support then hire a coach. Investing in yourself is very important and you deserve it all. Woop, woop...let's do this!

ABOUT THE AUTHOR

Margaret LeDane is an author and certified health coach for motivated and passionate people.

Over the years, she has dedicated her life to sharing the principles found in *Your A.W.E.S.O.M.E. Life: How to Reach Your Healthy Weight and Live Your Life Feeling Energized and Balanced* to help people find their healthy weight and live their dream-life.

Margaret speaks publicly and works virtually with private and group clients.

With her slow, steady approach to wellness, Margaret's clients enjoy huge successes in a manner that's relaxed and non-stressful.

In addition to her experience and professional training as a coach, Margaret earned a bachelor's degree in biology from Randolph-Macon Woman's College in Lynchburg, Virginia.

Margaret lives and works in the beautiful town of Annapolis, Maryland, the sailing capital of the world, with her two children and lovable pitbull mix dog, Bauer.

For fun she loves to Zumba, ride her bike, walk, hike, sail, travel and spend time with family and friends.

To learn more visit www.margaretledane.com/.

You can contact her at margaret@mybalancedbloodsugar.com or by phone at 410-533-0573.

SPECIAL OFFER FROM MARGARET!

If you enjoyed *Your A.W.E.S.O.M.E. Life: How to Reach Your Healthy Weight and Live Your Life Feeling Energized and Balanced*, please take a moment to sign up for her email list on her website https://www.margaretledane.com/ so you can continue to receive free tips on how to reach your healthy weight and live your dream-life.

Printed in Great Britain
by Amazon